Pressure Cooker Breakfast for Busy People

Mouth-Watering, and Easy To Follow Breakfast Recipes

Danielle Sanders

Sommario

Introduction

Considering the principle of diet in current times are based upon fasting, instead our keto instant pot is based upon the extreme decrease of carbs.

This kind of diet is based on the intake of specific foods that allow you to slim down faster permitting you to slim down approximately 3 kg each week.

You will certainly see how simple it will be to make these tasty meals with the tools available as well as you will certainly see that you will certainly be satisfied.

If you are reluctant concerning this fantastic diet plan you simply have to try it as well as analyze your results to a short time, trust me you will be pleased.

Bear in mind that the most effective method to reduce weight is to analyze your situation with the help of a specialist.

Blueberry Cheesecake Ice Cream

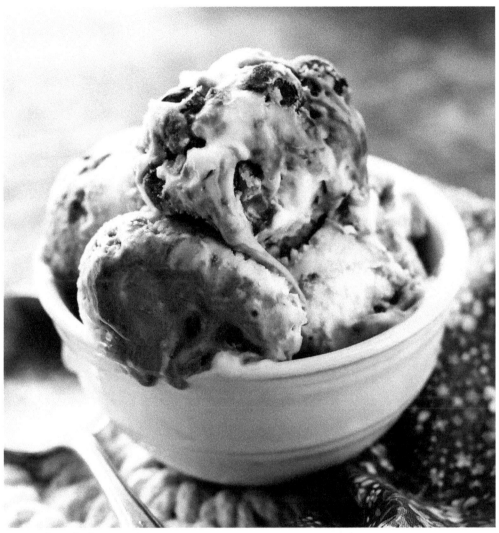

Ingredients for 6-8 servings:

2 cups whole milk 8 ounces reduced-fat cream cheese 3.4 ounce instant vanilla or cheesecake flavored pudding mix 3 tablespoons sugar 1 ½ cup frozen blueberries Crumbled graham crackers

Directions and total time – 60-90 m

• Seat glass pitcher on the base of the Instant Pot Ace and add milk, cream cheese, pudding mix, sugar, and frozen blueberries, in that order. • Secure and lock lid. • Choose the Frozen Desserts program (00:49 seconds). • Once program has completed, transfer ice cream to a freezer-safe container. • Cover and freeze until your desired consistency, about 2 hours for soft-serve consistency. If fully frozen, transfer to the fridge for 30 minutes to soften before scooping. • Serve topped with crumbled graham crackers to mimic a cheesecake's crust.

Raspberry Baked Oatmeal Bars
Ingredients for 6 servings:

3 cups steel cut oats 3 large eggs 2 cups unsweetened vanilla almond milk ⅓ cup erythritol ¼ tsp salt 1 cup frozen raspberries 1 tsp pure vanilla extract

Directions and total time – 15-30 m

• In a medium bowl, mix together all ingredients except the raspberries. Once the ingredients are well combined, fold in the raspberries. • Spray a 6" cake pan with cooking oil. Transfer the oat mixture to the pan and cover the pan with aluminum foil. • Pour 1 cup water into the Instant Pot and place the steam rack inside. Place the pan with the oat mixture on top of the rack. Secure the lid. • Press the Manual or Pressure Cook button and adjust the time to 15 minutes. • When the timer beeps, quick-release pressure until float valve drops and then unlock lid. • Carefully remove the pan from the inner pot and remove the foil. Allow to cool completely before cutting into bars and serving.

Fruity Quinoa & Granola Bowls
Ingredients for 4 servings:
1 cup quinoa rinsed 1 ½ cups Water 2 tbsp maple syrup plus more for topping (optional) 1 tsp vanilla extract ½ tsp ground cinnamon Pinch salt ½ - 1 cup nondairy milk 2 cups granola any variety 2 cups Fresh Fruit Compote Sliced bananas for topping (optional) Toasted walnuts for topping (optional)
Directions and total time – 15 m
• In your Instant Pot, combine the quinoa, water, maple syrup, vanilla, cinnamon, and salt. Lock the lid and turn the steam release handle to Sealing. Using the Manual or Pressure Cook function, set the cooker to High Pressure for 8 minutes (7 minutes at sea level). • When the cook time is complete, let the pressure release naturally for 10 minutes; quick release any remaining pressure. • Carefully remove the lid and stir the quinoa. Add enough milk to get the desired consistency. Spoon the quinoa mix into bowls and top with granola, compote, and any additional toppings, as desired.

Broccoli And Cheddar Crustless Quiche
Ingredients for 6 servings:
Nonstick cooking spray 1 cup Water 8 eggs ½ cup low-fat milk ½ cup whole wheat flour 1 cup chopped broccoli florets 1 ½ cups shredded Cheddar cheese divided ¼ tsp fine sea salt ¼ tsp freshly ground black pepper

Directions and total time – 30-60 m
• Spray an 8-inch ceramic soufflé dish with the cooking spray. • Place the trivet in the inner pot, then pour in the water. • If needed, make an aluminum sling. • In a large bowl, whisk together the eggs, milk, flour, broccoli, 1 cup of the cheese, and the salt and pepper. • Pour the mixture into the soufflé dish. Use the sling to lower the soufflé dish onto the trivet. • Lock the lid into place. Select Pressure Cook or Manual; set the pressure to High and the time to 30 minutes. Make sure the steam release knob is in the sealed position. After cooking, naturally release the pressure for 10 minutes, then quick release any remaining pressure. • Unlock and remove the lid. Use the sling to remove the soufflé dish. • Sprinkle the remaining ½ cup of cheese on top of the quiche. Using a sharp knife, slice the quiche into 6 wedges. Serve immediately, or place the quiche in an airtight container and refrigerate for up to 4 days.

Baked Oatmeal
Ingredients for 8-12 servings:
2 tbsp butter ½ cup brown sugar 2 eggs 1 cup peanut butter 1 cup milk 1 tsp Vanilla 3 cups quick-cooking oats 2 tsp baking powder ½ tsp salt ½ cup chocolate chips Powdered sugar for garnish optional
Directions and total time – 1-2 h
• In a medium bowl, beat together butter and sugar. Add eggs one at a time and beat until uniform. • Add peanut butter, milk and vanilla and stir to combine. • In a large bowl, stir together oats, baking powder and salt. Add wet ingredients and mix until fully incorporated. • Fold in chocolate chips. • Coat the inside of a 7 inch baking pan or casserole with nonstick spray • Spread batter in pan and cover pan with foil. • Pour one cup of water in the Instant Pot and insert the steam rack. Carefully lower the pan or casserole on to the steam rack, then secure the lid, making sure the vent is closed. • Using the display panel select the MANUAL or PRESSURE COOK function. Use the +/- keys and program the Instant Pot for 45 minutes. • When the time is up, let the pressure naturally release for 15 minutes, then quick-release the remaining pressure. • Carefully remove the pan and allow to cool for 10 minutes before serving. • Garnish with powdered sugar (optional). Keep covered and serve all week for a quick breakfast or snack.

Steel-Cut Oatmeal with Cranberries and Almonds

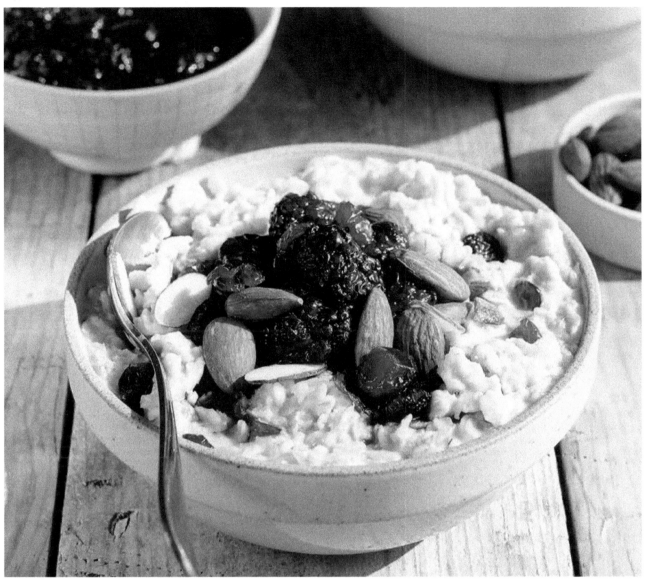

Ingredients for 2 servings:

1 tbsp unsalted butter ½ cup steel cut oats Pinch kosher salt 2 tsp sugar 1 cup Water ½ cup whole milk ¼ tsp vanilla extract ¼ cup dried cranberries ¼ cup toasted chopped almonds

Directions and total time – 30-60 m

• Select Sauté and adjust to Medium heat. Add the butter to the inner pot. When the butter has melted and stopped foaming, add the oats and stir to coat with the butter. Continue cooking for 2 to 3 minutes, or until the oats have a nutty aroma. • Add the salt, sugar, water, milk, vanilla, and cranberries. Stir to combine. • Lock the lid into place. Select Pressure Cook or Manual, and adjust the pressure to High and the time to 10 minutes. After cooking, let the pressure release naturally for 10 minutes, then quick release any remaining pressure. • Unlock the lid. Spoon the oatmeal into two bowls and top with the almonds. Adjust to your taste, adding extra milk or sugar if you like. Double It: Oatmeal is a great recipe for doubling, since the leftovers keep well for a couple of days in the refrigerator. Double all the ingredients and increase the salt to ¼ teaspoon. Cook time remains the same.

Cheddar-Herbed Strata
Ingredients for 4 servings:

6 eggs 1 cup full-fat Cheddar cheese shredded 1 cup spinach chopped ½ tbsp salted grass-fed butter softened 4 oz onion (¼ small onion) thinly sliced ½ tsp freshly ground black pepper ½ tsp kosher salt ½ tsp Dijon mustard ½ tsp paprika ½ tsp cayenne pepper ½ tsp cilantro dried ½ tsp sage dried ½ tsp parsley dried

Directions and total time –30-60 m

• Pour 1 cup of filtered water into the inner pot of the Instant Pot, then insert the trivet. In a large bowl, combine the eggs, cheese, spinach, butter, onion, black pepper, salt, mustard, paprika, cayenne pepper, cilantro, sage, and parsley. Mix thoroughly. Transfer this mixture into a wellgreased, Instant Pot–friendly dish. • Using a sling if desired, place the dish onto the trivet, and cover loosely with aluminum foil. Close the lid, set the pressure release to Sealing, and select Manual/Pressure Cook. Set the Instant Pot to 40 minutes on high pressure and let cook. • Once cooked, let the pressure naturally disperse from the Instant Pot for about 10 minutes, then carefully switch the pressure release to Venting. • Open the Instant Pot and remove the dish. Let cool, serve, and enjoy!

Bacon Quiche

Ingredients for 4 servings:

4 slices bacon cooked and crumbled ½ cup ham diced 1 + ⅓ cup sharp Cheddar cheese shredded (divided) 2 large green onions sliced thin 6 large eggs beaten ½ cup milk 1 cup Water Additional green onion for garnish optional

Directions and total time –30-60 m

• Mix together the meats, 1 cup cheese and green onion in the bottom of a 1,5 quart ovenproof casserole • In a large bowl, thoroughly whisk together eggs and milk. Pour egg mixture over meat mixture and stir to combine. Cover loosely with foil-do not seal. • Pour one cup of water in the Instant Pot and insert the steam rack. Use a foil sling to carefully lower the casserole on to the steam rack. • Secure the lid, making sure the vent is closed. • Using the display panel select the MANUAL or PRESSURE COOK function. Use the +/- keys and program the Instant Pot for 30 minutes. • When the time is up, let the pressure naturally release for 10 minutes, then quick-release the remaining pressure. • Carefully remove the casserole and top with remaining ⅓ cup cheese. Set under the broiler for 3-5 minutes until cheese begins to brown lightly. Serve immediately.

Breakfast Burritos
Ingredients for 8 servings:
Egg Mixture: 6 eggs ¼ cup milk ¼ cup sour cream ½ cup shredded Cheddar cheese 1 tsp onion salt ⅛ tsp pepper 2 ½ cups frozen hash browns 1 cup diced ham 1 cup fresh spinach chopped (optional) 12 6 flour tortillas warmed, "fajita size"

Directions and total time –30-60 m
• In a medium bowl, whisk the Egg Mixture ingredients until thoroughly incorporated. Set aside. • Coat the inside of a 1.5 qt casserole with non-stick spray. • Layer hash browns then ham in an even layer in the casserole dish. Pour egg mixture over the top. Cover with foil. • Pour one cup of water in the Instant Pot and insert the trivet. Carefully lower the casserole on to the trivet, then secure the lid, making sure the vent is closed. • Using the display panel select the MANUAL or PRESSURE COOK function. Use the +/- keys and program the Instant Pot for 25 minutes. • When the time is up, quick-release the remaining pressure. Open the pot and rinse the inside of the lid in cold water to help it reseal. • Add the chopped fresh spinach, stir, then replace the foil. Secure the lid, making sure the vent is closed. • Using the display panel select the MANUAL or PRESSURE COOK function. Use the +/- keys and program the Instant Pot for 10 minutes. • When the time is up, quick-release the remaining pressure. • Divide the egg mixture among the tortillas, roll and serve immediately, or store for up to 4 days in the refrigerator in a tightly sealed container. Reheat for 30 seconds in the microwave for a quick on-the-go breakfast.

Mini Mushroom Quiche
Ingredients for 6 servings:

3 ounces asiago cheese shredded 2 ounces mushrooms finely diced 1 tbsp chives snipped 3 tbsp spinach leaves cut into thin ribbons 4 eggs beaten ¼ cup heavy cream or half and half ½ tsp garlic salt ½ tsp kosher salt 1 cup Water Additional asiago cheese for garnish (optional)

Directions and total time –15-30 m

• Coat the inside of a silicone mold with nonstick spray • Firmly press the asiago cheese into the bottom and slightly up the sides of the silicone mold. Top with diced mushrooms, chives and spinach. • Combine the eggs, cream, garlic salt and salt in a medium bowl and whisk thoroughly. Pour into molds. Molds should not be more than ¾ full. • Pour 1 cup of water in the Instant Pot and insert the trivet. Carefully lower the mold on to the trivet. Secure the lid, making sure the vent is closed. • Using the display panel select the MANUAL or PRESSURE COOK function. Use the +/- buttons and program the Instant Pot for 5 minutes. • When the time is up, let the pressure naturally release for 5 minutes, then quick-release the remaining pressure. • Carefully remove the mold and turn out onto a plate while still warm. Immediately flip each mini quiche so that the mushrooms are on top and press down lightly with fingers to flatten the bottom of each quiche. • Garnish with additional asiago cheese if desired. Serve warm.

Crustless Artichoke and Olive Quiche
Ingredients for 6 servings:
6 large eggs ¼ cup whole milk 2 tsp chopped fresh dill ½ tsp salt ¼ tsp
ground black pepper 1 Roma Tomato seeded and diced ¼ cup diced jarred
artichokes drained ¼ cup sliced pitted Kalamata olives ¼ cup crumbled feta
cheese ¼ cup peeled and diced red onion 2 cups Water
Directions and total time –15-30 m
• In a medium bowl, whisk eggs, milk, dill, salt, and pepper. Stir in tomato,
artichokes, olives, feta cheese, and onion. Set aside. • Add egg mixture to a
7-cup glass dish greased with either oil or cooking spray. • Add water to the
Instant Pot. Insert steam rack. Place dish with egg mixture on steam
rack. Lock lid. • Press the Manual or Pressure Cook button and adjust cook
time to 8 minutes. When timer beeps, let pressure release naturally for 10
minutes. Quick-release any additional pressure until float valve drops and
then unlock lid. • Remove dish from pot and let sit 10 minutes. Slice and
serve warm.

French Toast Casserole with Peach

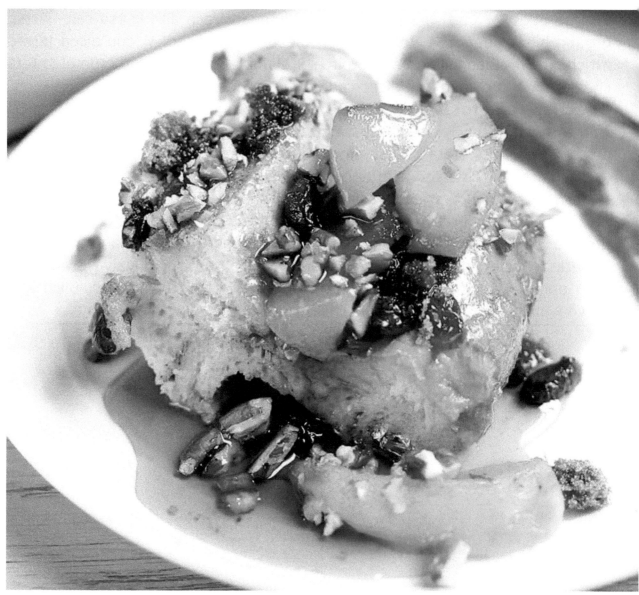

Ingredients for 4 servings:

4 tsp unsalted butter divided 6 slices whole grain bread cut into ½-inch cubes (about 4 cups) 2 large eggs 1 cup whole milk ½ tsp ground cinnamon ¾ cup packed-in-juice canned peaches 2 tbsp pecans chopped 1 tsp confectioners' sugar 4 tbsp maple syrup

Directions and total time – 30-60 m • Place the steam rack in the inner pot and add 1 cup water to the bottom of the pot. • Coat the interior of a 1-quart (1l) soufflé dish with 1 teaspoon of the butter and then add the bread cubes to the dish. • In a medium bowl, combine the eggs, milk, and cinnamon. Whisk to combine, and then add the peaches and canning juice.

Stir to combine. • Pour the egg mixture over the bread cubes and gently press the cubes into egg mixture until thoroughly coated in the mixture. • Cut the remaining butter into small pieces and evenly distribute over top of the bread cubes. Loosely cover the soufflé dish with aluminum foil. • Cover, lock the lid, and flip the steam release handle to the sealing position. Select Pressure Cook (Low) and set the cook time for 30 minutes. When the cook time is complete, quick release the pressure. • Open the lid. Carefully transfer the dish to a cooling rack and let the casserole cool for 10 minutes. • Garnish with the pecans and dust with the confectioners' sugar. Cut into 4 equal-sized portions and then drizzle 1 tablespoon maple syrup over top of each portion just before serving. Serve warm.

Yogurt Soy Milk Powder

 Ingredients for 4-6 servings:

 2 ½ cups hot water ¾ cup soy milk powder 1 teaspoon sugar ¾ teaspoon agar powder ¼ teaspoon probiotic or vegan starter culture

Directions and total time – more than 2 h • Add water, soy milk powder and sugar to a high-speed blender. Blend for 3 minutes (The temperature will be around 166°F) • Add the agar powder and blend for 30 seconds longer (the temperature will now be around 172°F) • Allow the soy milk to cool down to 110°F (you can speed this process up by placing the blender carafe into a bowl of ice water). • Once the temperature is down to 110°F, add the probiotic powder or vegan culture and whisk into the soy milk (don't blend it) • Pour the soy milk into two 16-ounce glass jars. • Close the Instant Pot, set to sealing, and select the "yogurt" setting for 14 hours. • Remove the jars from the multi cooker, cover with lids, and allow to cool on the counter before storing in the refrigerator. Though firm out of the Instant Pot, this is best served after two or more hours in the refrigerator. Enjoy!

Cardamom Yogurt with Roasted Peaches

Ingredients for 3 servings: For the yogurt: 8 cups whole milk 10 green cardamom pods lightly crushed 2 tablespoons plain yogurt ¼ cup granulated sugar 1 teaspoon ground cardamom ½ teaspoon vanilla extract 6 peaches halved and pitted 6 tablespoons old-fashioned rolled oats 3 tablespoons unsalted butter melted 2 tablespoons firmly packed brown sugar ¼ teaspoon ground cardamom

Directions and total time – more than 2 h • To make the yogurt, pour the milk into the Instant Pot. Enclose the cardamom pods in a square of cheesecloth and add to the pot. • Lock the lid in place and turn the valve to Sealing. Press the Yogurt button until the screen says boil and cook until the milk reaches 180°F, about 25 minutes. • Have ready an ice-water bath. Remove the lid and check the milk temperature with an instantread thermometer. If it is not 180°F, press the Keep Warm/Cancel program to reset the program, then select Sauté and heat until it reaches 180°F. Remove and discard the cardamom. • Transfer the inner pot to the ice-water bath, then stir the milk until it cools to 110°F, about 10 minutes. Transfer 1 cup of the milk to a small bowl, whisk in the yogurt until smooth, then return the milk-yogurt mixture to the pot and add the granulated sugar, cardamom, and vanilla. Whisk until blended. • Return the inner pot to the Instant Pot housing. Lock the lid in place; the valve can be turned to Sealing or Venting. Press the Keep Warm/Cancel button to reset the program, then press the Yogurt button and set the cook time for 10 hours. When the yogurt is ready (the screen will read Yogt), remove the lid, use pot holders to lift out the inner pot, cover it with plastic wrap, and refrigerate until the yogurt sets, about 4 hours. Do not stir at this point. • When the yogurt is set, line a large fine-mesh sieve with 4 layers of cheesecloth, place the sieve over a bowl, spoon the yogurt into the sieve, and refrigerate for 2 hours to drain. • Meanwhile, prepare the roasted peaches. Preheat the oven to 350°F. Butter a 9-inch square baking dish. • Arrange the peaches, cut side up, in the prepared dish. In a small bowl, stir together oats, butter, brown sugar, and cardamom, mixing well. Sprinkle the oat mixture evenly over the peaches. Roast in the oven until the peaches are juicy and tender and the topping is browned, 30–35 minutes. • To serve, spoon the yogurt into individual bowls and top with the peaches.

Bacon and Egg Breakfast Pastry
Ingredients for 4 servings:
8 oz sheet frozen puff pastry ⅔ cup shredded cheese 4 slices of bacon cooked and crumbled 4 eggs Finely chopped parsley or chives for garnish

Directions and total time – 15-30 m
• Follow the package directions for thawing and unfolding the puff pastry on a lightly floured surface. • Cut pastry into 4 squares. Place 2 squares on a cooking tray. • Place the drip pan in the bottom of the cooking chamber. Using the display panel, select AIRFRY, then adjust the temperature to 390 degrees and the time to 10 minutes for over easy (or up to 15 minutes for thoroughly cooked eggs), then touch START. • When the display indicates "Add Food" insert the cooking tray in the center position. • After 5 minutes, removed the pastry from the cooking chamber. Use a metal spoon to press down the center of each pastry to make a "nest", being careful not to collapse the sides. • Sprinkle ¼ of the cheese into each depression and push it to the side to line the nest. • Sprinkle ¼ of the cooked bacon around the edges of the nest. • Carefully crack an egg into each of the nests and return the tray to the cooking chamber. • When the display indicates "Turn Food" do nothing. • When cooking time is complete, check the eggs for desired doneness. • Repeat with the other half of pastry. Serve warm garnished with chopped parsley or chives.

Pumpkin Pie Custard
Ingredients for 6 servings:
2 cups fresh pumpkin puree or 2 cans pure pumpkin 15-ounce 6 egg 1 cup full fat coconut milk ¾ cup pure maple syrup or light-colored raw honey 1 tablespoon Pumpkin Pie Spice ¾ teaspoon finely grated lemon zest 2 teaspoons pure vanilla extract ¼ teaspoon sea salt

Directions and total time – 20-30 m
• Whisk together the pumpkin puree, eggs, coconut milk, maple syrup, pumpkin pie spice, lemon zest, vanilla extract, and sea salt. Divide the mixture evenly into 6 ramekins. • Place 2 cups of lukewarm water into the Instant Pot and place the wire rack at the bottom. • Cover the ramekins tightly with silicone lids or foil. Place them on the wire rack. • Turn the Instant Pot to manual or pressure cook high pressure and set it for 6 minutes. Hit the cancel button and let the machine naturally release the pressure, about 15 to 20 minutes. Remove the ramekins, uncover them to the condensation doesn't build up, and allow them to cool completely on a wire rack. Cover the ramekins with plastic wrap and place the ramekins in the refrigerator for up to 5 days.

Cornmeal Porridge
Ingredients for 4 servings:
1 cup fine cornmeal 1 can coconut milk, full fat 4 ½ cups water ½ cup organic cane sugar 1 teaspoon vanilla ¼ teaspoon ground nutmeg ¼ teaspoon cinnamon ½ teaspoon salt

Directions and total time – 15 m
• Press the Saute button on your Instant Pot. Place water, coconut milk, cornmeal and sugar in the Instant Pot and stir using a whisk so there are no lumps. • Bring mixture to a simmer and whisk again. Put the lid on the Instant Pot and set the pressure release valve to Sealing. Cancel the Saute function, Press the Manual or Pressure Cook button then select the + button to set the timer for 9 minutes. • At the end of the cycle, press the off Mode and let the pot natural release for 10 minutes. Turn the valve to Venting to manual or quick release the remaining steam. • Once the pin in the lid drops, open the lid, stir the porridge. Add traditional spices, vanilla, cinnamon, nutmeg and salt or vanilla, cardamon, and coriander and serve.

Amaranth Porridge

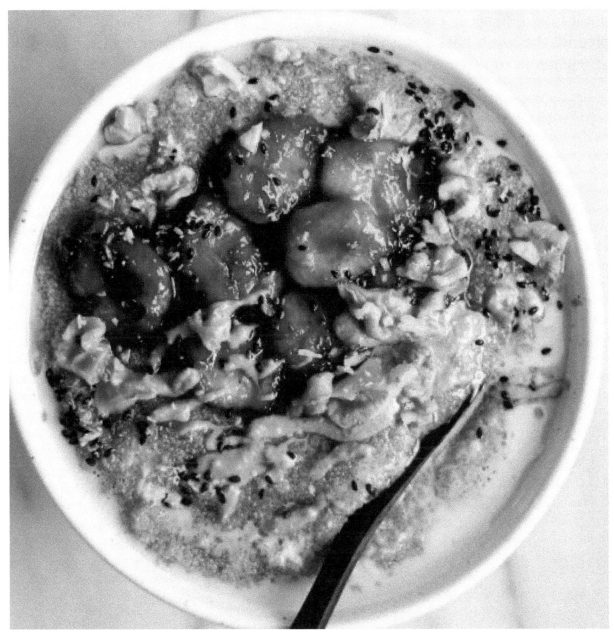

Ingredients for 2 servings:
2 cup uncooked amaranth 5 cup unsweetened almond milk 4 ripe bananas, sliced 1 teaspoon ground cinnamon, for topping 4 scoops collagen peptides or your favorite protein powder (optional, for extra protein)

Directions and total time – 30 m
• For pressure cooker: Combine amaranth, almond milk, and bananas into a 3-quart pressure cooker. Cook on high pressure for 5 minutes and let the pressure come down naturally for at least 10 minutes. Serve hot with

cinnamon sprinkled on top and collagen peptides stirred in. ● For stove-top cooking: Bring almond milk to a gentle boil in a lidded pot. Stir in the amaranth and sliced bananas, lower the heat, and simmer for 25-30 minutes, or until the grain has absorbed most of the liquid. Serve hot with cinnamon sprinkled on top (porridge will thicken as it sits).

Hard Boiled Eggs
Ingredients for 2 servings:

12 eggs 1 cup water

Directions and total time – 20 m

• Place the steaming rack in the bottom of a 6-quart Instant Pot. Pour in the water, then arrange the eggs in an even layer on the rack. Cover and set the valve to "sealing." • Set to cook on "Manual" high pressure for 5 minutes. Once the timer goes off, wait another 3 minutes (the timer should begin counting back up as the pressure naturally releases). Then carefully set the valve to "venting" to quick-release the remaining pressure. (I recommend placing a towel over the vent when you first turn the valve to cover the steam. • Once all of the pressure has vented, remove the lid and carefully transfer the eggs to an ice bath (a bowl filled with water and lots of ice) for 5 minutes to cool the eggs down. • Peel and enjoy immediately. Or refrigerate the peeled eggs in a sealed container for up to 1 week.

Lentils and Poached Eggs
Ingredients for 4 servings:

¾ cup dried brown or green lentils, rinsed and drained 2 dried bay leaves 3 cups Water divided 3 tbsp extra-virgin olive oil 1 tbsp finely chopped fresh parsley 1 lemon Grated zest and juice ½ tsp salt divided Nonstick cooking spray 4 eggs 4 cups baby spinach ¼ tsp black pepper

Directions

and total time – 30-60 m • Place the lentils, bay leaves, and 2 cups of the water in the Instant Pot. Seal the lid, close the valve, and set the Manual/Pressure Cook button to 7 minutes. • Meanwhile, in a small bowl, whisk together the oil, parsley, lemon zest and juice, and ¼ tsp of the salt. Set aside. • Coat 4 (6 oz) ramekins with cooking spray and crack 1 egg into each ramekin. Set aside. • Use a quick pressure release. When the valve drops, carefully remove the lid and drain the lentils (discarding the lentil water and 2 bay leaves). Return the lentils to the Instant Pot with the spinach and ¼ tsp of the salt. Toss until the spinach is just wilted and divide it between 4 soup bowls. Cover to keep warm. • Add 1 cup of water to the pot, add a trivet and 3 ramekins. Stack the 4th ramekin on top of the other ramekins. Seal the lid, close the valve, press the Cancel button, and reset the Manual/Pressure Cook button to 1 minute. • Use a natural pressure release for 1 minute, followed by a quick pressure release. When the valve drops, carefully remove the lid. Remove the ramekins and drain off any excess water that may have accumulated while cooking. Carefully run a knife around the outer edges of each egg to release from the ramekin easily. • Spoon equal amounts of the oil mixture on top of each serving of lentils and top with the eggs. Sprinkle with black pepper.

Broccoli-Cheddar Egg Muffins
Ingredients for 7 servings:
3 large eggs ¾ ounce wedge Laughing Cow light Swiss cheese OR 1 ½ tablespoons cream cheese 1 cup broccoli florets chopped 1 green onion white and green parts, thinly sliced ¼ cup shredded Cheddar cheese

Directions and total time – 15 m
• In a wide mouthed 1-pint Mason jar, combine the eggs and Laughing Cow cheese. Using an immersion blender, blend for about 15 seconds, just until smooth. • Pour 1 cup water into the Instant Pot. Generously grease 7 silicone muffin cups with butter, making sure to coat all of the ridges well. Place the muffin cups on a long-handled silicone steam rack. • Sprinkle the broccoli and green onions among the muffin cups, then pour in the egg mixture, dividing it evenly and filling each cup about half full. Sprinkle the cups evenly with the Cheddar cheese. Holding the handles of the steam rack, carefully lower the muffin cups into the pot. If necessary, clasp together the handles of the steam rack. • Secure the lid and set the Pressure Release to Sealing. Select the Steam setting and set the cooking time for 8 minutes at low pressure. (The pot will take about 5 minutes to come up to pressure before the cooking program begins.) • When the cooking program ends, let the pressure release naturally for 5 minutes, then move the Pressure Release to Venting to release any remaining steam. Open the pot. The egg muffins will have puffed up quite a bit during cooking, but they will deflate and settle as they cool. Wearing heat-resistant mitts, grasp the handles of the steam rack and lift the muffin cups out of the pot. Let the muffins cool for about 5 minutes, until you are able to comfortably handle them. • To unmold, pull the sides of the muffin cups away from the muffins and transfer the muffins to plates. Serve warm.

Sausage and Egg Sandwiches
Ingredients for 4 servings:

4 large eggs 2 tbsp whole milk ¼ tsp salt ⅛ tsp black pepper 1 ½ cups Water 4 English muffins 2 tsp butter 4 breakfast sausage patties Cheddar cheese slices 4 slices

Directions and total time – 15-30 m

• Spray four ramekins with cooking spray and set aside. • In a small bowl, whisk together eggs, milk, salt, and pepper. Pour evenly into four ramekins. Wrap ramekins tightly in foil. • Pour 1 ½ cups water into Instant Pot. • Place foil-wrapped ramekins into Instant Pot, stacked two by two. Close lid and set pressure release to Sealing. • Press Manual or Pressure Cook button and adjust time to 8 minutes. • While eggs are cooking, toast English muffins and spread with butter. • When the timer beeps, let pressure release naturally for 2 minutes and then quick release the remaining pressure. Unlock lid and remove it. • Carefully remove ramekins from Instant Pot. Pour out water from cooking pot and put cooking pot back into Instant Pot. • Press Sauté button and place sausage patties inside Instant Pot. Heat sausage patties, turning once, 1 minute. Remove from Instant Pot. • Remove each egg from its ramekin and place on one half of English muffin. Top each egg with a sausage patty and a slice of cheese. Place other half of the English muffin on top to create a sandwich.

Spinach and Feta Frittata
Ingredients for 6 servings:
6 eggs beaten ¾ cup half and half ½ cup sour cream 2 tsp Dijon mustard ½ tsp pepper 3 oz feta cheese crumbled ¼ cup diced green onions 3 cups chopped baby spinach ½ cup bacon crumbles optional spinach cut in ribbons, for garnish

Directions and total time – 30-60 m
• In a large bowl, whisk together beaten eggs, half and half, sour cream, dijon and pepper. • Add remaining ingredients and stir to combine. • Coat the inside of a 1.5 qt oven-proof casserole with nonstick spray and fill with egg mixture. Cover loosely with foil--do not seal. • Pour one cup of water in the Instant Pot and insert the steam rack. Use a foil sling to carefully lower the casserole on to the steam rack. • Secure the lid, making sure the vent is closed. • Using the display panel select the MANUAL function. Use the +/- keys and program the Instant Pot for 30 minutes. • When the time is up, let the pressure naturally release for 10 minutes, then quick-release the remaining pressure. • Carefully remove the casserole. Serve hot garnished with additional spinach cut in ribbons.

Best Fruity Quinoa

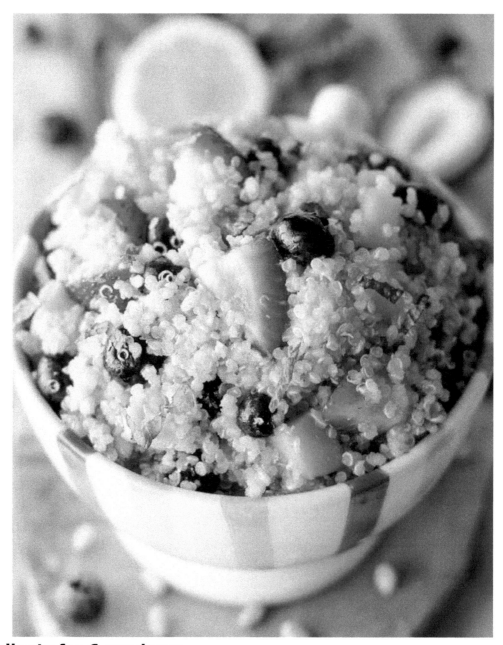

Ingredients for 6 servings:
3 ½ lb assorted sweet and tart apples 2 tsp lemon juice freshly squeezed 2 tsp ghee ¼ tsp ground cinnamon plus more for serving ⅛ tsp ground allspice ⅛ tsp fine sea salt

Directions and total time – 15-30 m

• Peel, core, and slice the apples. Place the apples, ¾ cup water, and the lemon juice, ghee, cinnamon, allspice, and salt in an electric pressure cooker. • If using an Instant Pot, secure the lid and turn the valve to pressure.

Select the Manual or Pressure Cook button and set it to high pressure for 5 minutes.Once the timer has sounded, let the machine release the pressure on its own; it will take about 15 minutes. (Alternatively, carefully release the pressure manually.) Remove the lid. • Using an immersion blender or conventional blender, pulse the applesauce to your desired consistency. Serve warm with cinnamon sprinkled on top, or refrigerate and enjoy chilled. • Store the applesauce in an airtight container in the refrigerator for 10 days or in an airtight container in the freezer for 6 months. Allow it to thaw overnight in the refrigerator before serving. If desired, reheat in a saucepan over medium-low heat for 8 to 10 minutes, until heated through.

Eggs "en Cocotte"
Ingredients for 2 servings:
1 tablespoon unsalted butter 1 teaspoon extra-virgin olive oil 4 white button or cremini mushrooms halved and sliced 1 tablespoon chopped onion ½ cup vegetable or Mushroom Stock ½ cup heavy cream whipping 1 tablespoon dry Sherry ½ teaspoon kosher salt Pinch freshly ground black pepper 2 large eggs 2 tablespoons grated sharp cheddar cheese 1 tablespoon chopped fresh chives to garnish

Directions and total time – 15 m
• Select Sauté and adjust to Medium heat. Add the butter and olive oil to the inner pot and heat until the butter is foaming. Add the mushrooms and cook, stirring occasionally, until they release their liquid, about 5 minutes. Add the onion and cook for about 4 minutes, or until soft. • Add the stock, cream, and sherry, and cook until the liquid has reduced by half, about 5 minutes. Stir in the salt and pepper. • Divide the mixture between two ramekins. Break an egg into each of the ramekins, and sprinkle each with the Cheddar cheese. • Rinse out the inner pot and return it to the base. Add 1 cup of water to the inner pot and place the trivet inside. Place the ramekins, uncovered, on the trivet. • Lock the lid into place. Select Pressure Cook or Manual, and adjust the pressure to High and time to 2 minutes (for runny yolks). After cooking, quick release the pressure. • Let the egg cups cool for a minute, and serve garnished with the chives.

Omelette Potatoes
Ingredients for 4 servings:
1 cup Water 2 lbs russet potatoes 4 potatoes total 3 eggs beaten ¼ cup diced ham 2 tbsp diced red onion 1 tbsp finely chopped parsley ¼ cup shredded cheese Salt and freshly ground pepper to taste
Directions and total time – 30-60 m
• Slice the top off each potato lengthwise. Each "lid" should be about ½ inch thick at its thickest point. (Discard "lids" or reserve for another use.) • Pour one cup of water in the Instant Pot and insert the steam rack. Place the potatoes on the rack. • Secure the lid, making sure the vent is closed. • Using the display panel select the MANUAL or PRESSURE COOK function. Use the +/- keys and program the Instant Pot for 12 minutes. • When the time is up, quick-release the pressure. • Carefully remove the potatoes from the pot to a cutting board and allow to cool slightly. • Scoop out the center of the potato flesh, being careful not to pierce the skin and to leave enough "structure" so the potato stands up easily on its own. • Roughly mash half the scooped out centers in a medium bowl. Don't worry if it's not completely cooked. • (Set aside the other half of the potato centers for some other use, or discard.) • Add eggs, ham, onion, parsley and 2 tbsp of the cheese to the potatoes and stir to combine. • Fill each potato shell with the egg mixture and top with remaining cheese. • Place the potatoes on the steam rack again, then secure the lid, making sure the vent is closed. • Using the display panel select the MANUAL or PRESSURE COOK function. Use the +/- keys and program the Instant Pot for 6 minutes. • When the time is up, quick-release the pressure. • (Optional) Set the potatoes under the broiler to brown the cheese. Serve hot topped with freshly ground pepper and a sprinkling of salt.

Bacon and Asiago Egg Bites

Ingredients for 4 servings:

4 eggs ¾ cup shredded asiago cheese ½ cup cottage cheese ¼ cup heavy cream ½ tsp salt ¼ tsp pepper 1 dash hot sauce optional 4 strips bacon cooked and crumbled

Directions and total time – 15-30 m

• Add all ingredients except the bacon to a blender. Blend until smooth (about 15 seconds). • Coat the inside of silicone egg mold with nonstick spray. • Evenly distribute the bacon into the egg molds. Pour egg mixture evenly over bacon and cover loosely with foil. • Pour one cup of water in the Instant Pot and insert the steam rack. • Carefully lower the egg mold onto the steam rack, then secure the lid, making sure the vent is closed. • Using the display panel select the MANUAL or PRESSURE COOK function. Use the +/- keys and program the Instant Pot for 10 minutes. • When the time is up, quick-release the pressure. Remove the egg mold and let cool for 2-3 minutes. • Unmold the egg bites and enjoy immediately or refrigerate up to one week.

Crustless Meat Lovers Quiche

Ingredients for 4 servings:

6 eggs 1 cup full-fat Cheddar cheese shredded 1 cup spinach chopped ½ tbsp salted grass-fed butter softened 4 oz onion (¼ small onion) thinly sliced ½ tsp freshly ground black pepper ½ tsp kosher salt ½ tsp Dijon mustard ½ tsp paprika ½ tsp cayenne pepper ½ tsp cilantro dried ½ tsp sage dried ½ tsp parsley dried

Directions and total time –30-60 m

• Pour 1 cup of filtered water into the inner pot of the Instant Pot, then insert the trivet. In a large bowl, combine the eggs, cheese, spinach, butter, onion, black pepper, salt, mustard, paprika, cayenne pepper, cilantro, sage, and parsley. Mix thoroughly. Transfer this mixture into a wellgreased, Instant Pot–friendly dish. • Using a sling if desired, place the dish onto the trivet, and cover loosely with aluminum foil. Close the lid, set the pressure release to Sealing, and select Manual/Pressure Cook. Set the Instant Pot to 40 minutes on high pressure and let cook. • Once cooked, let the pressure naturally disperse from the Instant Pot for about 10 minutes, then carefully switch the pressure release to Venting. • Open the Instant Pot and remove the dish. Let cool, serve, and enjoy!

Strawberry Jam
Ingredients for 2 servings:
 4 cups strawberries hulled and quartered 1 ½ cups sugar 3 tbsp lemon juice 3 tbsp Water 3 tbsp cornstarch
Directions and total time –30-60 m
• Mix together strawberries and sugar in the Instant Pot. Set aside for 30 minutes to allow the berries to macerate (soften and release juices). • After 30 minutes, add lemon juice and stir to combine. • Secure the lid, making sure the vent is closed. • Using the display panel select the MANUAL or PRESSURE COOK function. Use the +/- keys and program the Instant Pot for 1 minute. • When the time is up, let the pressure naturally release for 15 minutes, then quick-release the remaining pressure. • Turn the pot off by selecting CANCEL, then select the SAUTÉ function. • In a small bowl, mix together cornstarch and cold water. Stir into the pot. Cook and stir until desired thickness is reached. • Turn the pot off and allow to cool.

Crispy Frittata Florentine

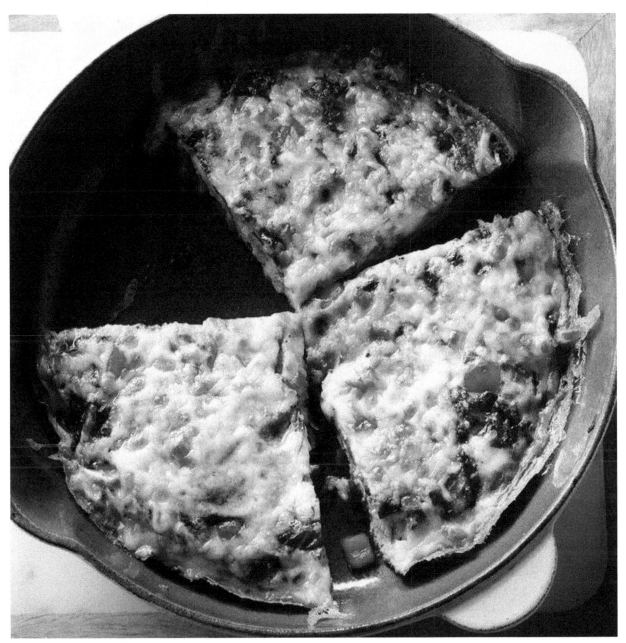

Ingredients for 4-6 servings:

4 slices bacon chopped 2 tbsp oil 2 cups frozen hash browns 5 eggs 2 tbsp half and half (or milk) 1 tsp mustard powder 1 tsp kosher salt 1 tsp kosher salt ⅔ cup fresh spinach finely chopped

Directions and total time −15-30 m

• In a medium bowl. whisk together eggs, half and half and spices. Stir in spinach and set aside. • Using the display panel select the SAUTE function. Add chopped bacon to the Instant Pot and cook until crisp. • Using a slotted spoon, remove bacon to a paper towel-lined plate. • Add frozen hash browns in an even layer and brown, without stirring, 6-8 minutes. • Drizzle with oil, then turn the hash browns in sections. Cook without stirring an additional 4-6 minutes. • Turn the pot off by selecting CANCEL. Remove hash browns to a plate, leaving any remaining drippings. • Pour in egg mixture and use a wooden spoon to scrape the brown bits from the bottom of the pot. • Return the hash browns to the pot and fold in gently, then sprinkle cooked bacon evenly over the top. • Secure the lid, making sure the vent is closed. • Using the display panel select the MANUAL or PRESSURE COOK function. Use the +/- keys and program the Instant Pot for 1 minute and adjust to LOW PRESSURE. • When the time is up, quick-release the remaining pressure. Cut frittata into wedges and serve warm.

Pina Colada Oatmeal
Ingredients for 4 servings:
1 tbsp coconut oil 2 cups coconut milk 1 cup pineapple juice 1 cup steel cut oats 1 ½ cups fresh pineapple diced ¾ cup sweetened shredded coconut raspberries or maraschino cherries for topping (optional)

Directions and total time −15-30 m
• Pour coconut oil, coconut milk, pineapple juice and oats into Instant Pot in that order. Swirl to make sure all oats are submerged. • Secure the lid, making sure the vent is closed. • Using the display panel select the MANUAL function. Use the +/- keys and program the Instant Pot for 3 minutes. • When the time is up, let the pressure release naturally until the pin drops (about 15 minutes). • Stir in coconut and pineapple. Serve with raspberries or maraschino cherries (optional).

Breakfast Hash
Ingredients for 4-6 servings:
3 tbsp butter 1 medium yellow onion chopped (1 cup) 1 medium green bell pepper stemmed, cored, and chopped (1 cup) 1 medium red bell pepper stemmed, cored, and chopped (1 cup) 1 lb smoked deli ham (not thinly shaved), any coating removed, the meat diced 2 medium garlic cloves peeled and minced (2 teaspoons) 1 tsp dried sage 1 tsp dried thyme ½ tsp celery seeds (optional) ¼ tsp fine table salt ¼ tsp ground black pepper 1 lb yellow potatoes diced (no need to peel) 1 ½ cups chicken broth

Directions and total time – 30-60 m
• Press Saute, set time for 5 minutes. • Melt the butter in the cooker. Add the onion and both bell peppers. Cook, stirring occasionally, until softened, about 4 minutes. Add the ham, garlic, sage, thyme, celery seeds (if using), salt, and pepper. Cook, stirring often, until fragrant, about 1 minute. • Turn off the SAUTE function. Stir in the potatoes and broth, scraping up any browned bits on the pot's bottom. Lock the lid onto the cooker. • Optional 1 Max Pressure Cooker Press Pressure cook on Max pressure for 10 minutes with the Keep Warm setting off. • Optional 2 All Pressure Cookers Press Pressure cook (Manual) on High pressure for 12 minutes with the Keep Warm setting off. • Use the quick-release method to bring the pot's pressure back to normal. Unlatch the lid and open the cooker. Stir well. • Press Saute, set time for 10 minutes. • Bring the mixture to a simmer, stirring often. Continue without stirring until the liquid boils off and the hash touching the hot surface starts to brown, 3 to 4 minutes. Turn off the SAUTE function and remove the hot insert from the machine to stop the cooking. Some of the potatoes may have fused to the surface. Use a metal spatula to get them up. The point is to have some browned bits and some softer bits throughout the hash.

Sausage and Kale Egg Muffins

Ingredients for 2 servings:

1 tsp avocado oil 2 tsp bacon fat (or more avocado oil) 4 ounces fully cooked chicken sausage diced 4 small kale leaves any variety, finely chopped ½ tsp kosher salt ½ tsp ground black pepper 4 large eggs ¼ cup heavy (whipping) cream or full-fat coconut milk 4 tbsp shredded white cheddar or swiss cheese optional 1 cup Water

Directions and total time – 15-30 m

• Use the 1 teaspoon avocado oil to grease the bottom and insides of four silicone muffin cups (preferred), ceramic ramekins, or half-pint mason jars. If you have a silicone egg bites mold, you can also use that for this recipe. • Set the Instant Pot to Sauté and melt the bacon fat. Add the sausage and sauté for 2 minutes. Add the chopped kale and ¼ teaspoon each of the salt and pepper. Sauté until the kale is wilted, 2 to 3 minutes longer. • Meanwhile, in a medium bowl, lightly beat together the eggs, cream, and remaining ¼ teaspoon each salt and pepper • Press Cancel. Divide the kale-sausage mixture among the four muffin cups. Pour the egg mixture evenly over the kale and sausage and stir lightly with a fork. If desired, top each with 1 tablespoon shredded cheese. Loosely cover the cups with foil or silicone lids. • Pour the water into the Instant Pot. Place the metal steam rack/trivet inside. Place the four muffin cups on top. • Secure the lid and set the steam release valve to Sealing. Press the Pressure Cook or Manual button and set the cook time to 5 minutes. • When the Instant Pot beeps, allow the pressure to release naturally for 10 minutes, then carefully switch the steam release valve to Venting. • Carefully remove the muffins from the Instant Pot. Serve hot or warm.

Vanilla Yogurt
Ingredients for 6 servings:
4 cups milk 2% 3.5 ounces vanilla yogurt 1 tablespoon sugar
Directions and total time – more than 2 h
• Bring milk to boil in a medium size non-stick pot on high heat (option to do this in the Instant Pot by using the Saute function on high temperature). • Cool to near room temperature. • Add yogurt and sugar. Stir to mix. Divide the mixture into 4 heat proof cups. (If you used the Instant Pot for these steps, clean out the Instant Pot, it will be used in the following steps.) • In the Instant Pot, add 5 cups water. Place the 4 heat proof cups into the inner pot. Close the lid and choose "Keep Warm" function for 15 minutes. • Let the pot stand for 10 hours closed. • Open the lid and take out yogurt. Cover with plastic wrap and chill a few hours before serving.

Avocado Toasts with Egg

Ingredients for 4 servings:

3 cups Water divided 4 large eggs 2 cups ice cubes 2 avocados peeled and roughly mashed 1 jalapeno seeded (if desired) and minced 3 tbsp light mayonnaise 3 tbsp lemon juice 1 tsp Dijon mustard ¼ tsp salt 4 oz multigrain Italian loaf bread cut diagonally into 12 thin slices and lightly toasted ½ cup diced tomato ¼ cup chopped fresh cilantro 2 tbsp minced red onion 1 lemon cut into 4 wedges

Directions and total time – 15-30 m

Place 1 cup of the water into the Instant Pot. Top with a steamer basket. Arrange the eggs in the steamer basket. Seal the lid, close the valve, and set the Manual/Pressure Cook button to 7 minutes. 2. Meanwhile, combine the remaining 2 cups of water with the ice cubes in a medium bowl and place near the Instant Pot. 3. In a small bowl, stir together the mashed avocado, jalapeño, mayonnaise, lemon juice, mustard, and salt. 4. Use a quick pressure release. When the valve drops, carefully remove the lid and place the eggs immediately into the ice water. Let stand for 3 minutes. 5. Peel the eggs and cut the eggs in half, discarding 4 of the egg yolk halves. Add the remaining egg yolk halves to the avocado mixture and mash until well blended (it will be slightly lumpy). Finely chop all of the egg whites and set aside. 6. Spread the avocado mixture on bread slices (dividing it evenly between the slices) and top with the chopped egg whites, tomato, cilantro, and onion. Serve with the lemon wedges to squeeze over all.

Cheesy Ham and Potato Casserole

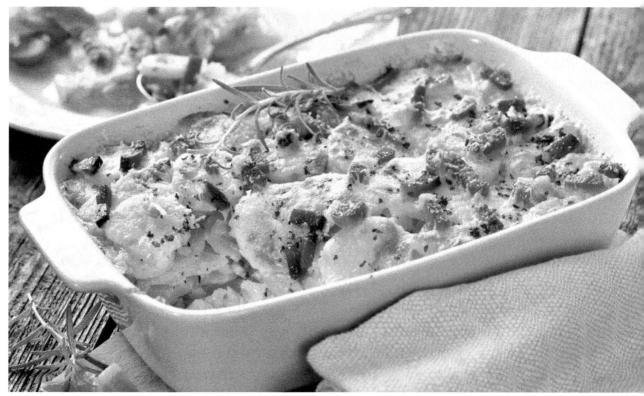

Ingredients for 4 servings:
1 cup chicken or beef broth 2 lbs frozen unseasoned hash brown cubes 2 frozen thin boneless ham steaks 8-ounces each 1 ½ tsp stemmed and minced sage leaves or ½ tsp dried sage 1 tsp stemmed thyme leaves or ½ tsp dried thyme 1 tsp onion powder ¼ tsp cayenne optional 2 cups Shredded Swiss or Cheddar cheese (8 ounces)

Directions and total time – 15-30 m
• Press the button SAUTÉ. Set it for MEDIUM, NORMAL, or CUSTOM 300°F and set the time for 5 minutes. • Pour the broth into an Instant Pot and heat it until wisps of steam rise off the liquid. (It can even come to a very low simmer— but not too much because you'll lose the liquid necessary for the pressure.) • Make an even layer of half the hash brown cubes in the pot. Turn off the SAUTÉ function. Break the ham steaks into thirds and set them on top of the potatoes. Make an even layer of the remaining potato cubes on the ham. Sprinkle the sage, thyme, onion powder, and cayenne (if using) evenly over the potatoes. Lock the lid onto the pot. • Option 1 Max Pressure Cooker Press Pressure cook on Max pressure for 3 minutes with the Keep Warm setting off. • Option 2 All Pressure Cookers Press Meat/Stew or Pressure cook (Manual) on High pressure for 4 minutes with the Keep Warm

setting off. The vent must be closed. • Use the quick-release method to bring the pot's pressure back to normal. Unlatch the lid and open the cooker. Sprinkle the cheese evenly over the top of the dish. Set the lid askew over the pot and set aside for 5 minutes to let the cheese melt before serving by the big spoonful

Purple Yam Barley Porridge
Ingredients for 12 servings:
3 tablespoons pearl barley 3 tablespoons pot barley 3 tablespoons buckwheat 3 tablespoons glutinous rice 3 tablespoons black glutinous rice 3 tablespoons black eye beans 3 tablespoons red beans 3 tablespoons romano beans 3 tablespoons brown rice 1 purple yam about 10.5 ounces ⅙ teaspoon baking soda optional

Directions and total time – 30-60 m
• Clean the purple yam, remove the skin and cut into 1 centimetre cubes. • Wash the barley, rice and beans in the inner pot of Instant Pot. • Place the purple yam and baking soda (if using) into the pot. • Add water up to the 8 cup mark on the inner pot. • Close the lid and put the steam release to the Sealing position. Select the [Porridge] program and keep pressing until the "More" setting is selected. • After the program finishes, let it cool for 10 minutes. Don't try to release the pressure as the starchy porridge will spill out. • Serve plain or with sugar, honey or blue agave syrup.

Millet Porridge
Ingredients for 2 servings:

⅓ cup millet 1 tablespoon brown sugar (you can use more or less) ½ teaspoon cinnamon ½ tablespoon unsalted butter 2 tablespoons raisins 1 cup milk Milk or cream for serving (optional) Frozen berries for serving (optional)

Directions and total time – 30 m

• Add 1 cup of cold water to your Instant Pot and place a trivet inside. • Add all the ingredients to a glass dish that fits into your Instant Pot, cover with foil and place on the trivet inside Instant Pot. • Close the lid of your Instant Pot and turn the valve to Sealing. • Press Manual or Pressure Cooker button (depending on your model) and use the arrows to select 12 minutes. It will take about 5-6 minutes to come to pressure. • Once the Instant Pot beeps that the 12 minutes of cooking are done, do natural pressure release for 10 minutes. It means that you do not touch your Instant Pot for 10 minutes and do nothing. • After 10 minutes of natural pressure release are done, do a quick release. This will take only a few seconds. • Very carefully, as it'll be really hot, remove the bowl with Millet Porridge from Instant Pot. • Open the foil and mix really well. If you notice that the milk is not fully absorbed, then cover with foil and let sit for another 3-5 minutes. • Transfer the cooked Millet Porridge to individual serving bowls, add a few splashes of milk or cream and garnish with fruit or frozen berries if desired. Enjoy hot!

Gingerbread Oatmeal and Buckweat Porridge
Ingredients for 6 servings:

¾ cup gluten-free steel cut oats ½ cup raw buckwheat groats, toasted on the stove until golden and fragrant 3-4 cups water or non-dairy milk or a combination (If making on the stovetop, dairy milk works) 3 tablespoons dark brown sugar 1 tablespoon dark molasses 1 teaspoon vanilla extract 1 teaspoon ground cinnamon ¾ teaspoon ground ginger ⅛ teaspoon ground cloves ¼ teaspoon salt For Serving Heavy cream, milk, or non-dairy milk Sliced pear Toasted pecans Toasted buckwheat groats

Directions and total time – 15-30 m

• If making in an Instant Pot, add all of the ingredients to the instant pot and stir to combine. Place the lid on the pot and make sure the pressure release valve is in the sealing position. Press the pressure cooker button, make sure it is on high, and set the timer for 6 minutes. When the timer is up, let the pressure cooker naturally release for 10 minutes. When the timer is up, release any additional pressure by carefully moving the pressure release valve into the venting position. • Bring the water or liquid to boil over medium high heat. Add all of the ingredients and stir well to combine. Reduce heat to a low simmer. Simmer, stirring occasionally, until most of the water has been absorbed to desired consistency and grains are cooked through, about 30 minutes. If your grains haven't cooked to your liking after the water has mostly been absorbed, add another 2 tablespoons of water at a time, until cooked through. • Serve warm with a splash of cream, sliced pears, toasted pecans, and buckwheat groats. • Store any leftovers in an airtight container in the refrigerator for up to a week. Add a few tablespoons of water to loosen it up while reheating.

Orzo with Herb and Lemon
Ingredients for 2 servings:

2 ½ cups dry orzo pasta ½ teaspoon sea salt 1 tablespoon dried parsley 1 teaspoon dried thyme 1 teaspoon dried garlic 1 teaspoon dried lemon zest 1 cup dehydrated peas 4 cups vegetable broth or water 2 tablespoons extra-virgin olive oil

Directions and total time – 15 m

• Layer the dry ingredients in the jar in the order listed. • Place all of the jarred ingredients into the Instant Pot. Add 4 cups of vegetable broth or water. Stir to mix. Cover with the lid and ensure the vent is in the "Sealed" position. Pressure Cook on High for 5 minutes. Allow the steam pressure to release naturally for 5 minutes, then release any remaining pressure manually.

Coconut Curry and Vegetable Rice Bowls
Ingredients for 6 servings:
⅔ cup uncooked brown rice rinsed and drained 1 cup Water 1 tsp curry powder ¾ tsp salt divided 1 cup chopped green onion both green and white parts 1 cup sliced red or yellow bell pepper 1 cup matchstick carrots 1 cup chopped red or purple cabbage 1 can sliced water chestnuts drained, 8 oz 1 can no salt added chickpeas rinsed and drained, 15 oz 1 can lite coconut milk 13 oz 1 tbsp grated fresh ginger 1 ½ tbsp sugar

Directions and total time – 30-60 m
• Combine the rice, water, curry powder, and ¼ tsp of the salt in the Instant Pot. • Seal the lid, close the valve, and set the Manual/Pressure Cook button to 15 minutes. • Use a natural pressure release for about 12 minutes. When the valve drops, carefully remove the lid and stir in the remaining ingredients. • Press the Cancel button and set to Sauté. Then press the Adjust button to "More" or "High." Bring to a boil and boil for 2 minutes, or until all the ingredients are heated through, stirring occasionally.

Creamy Carrot Soup

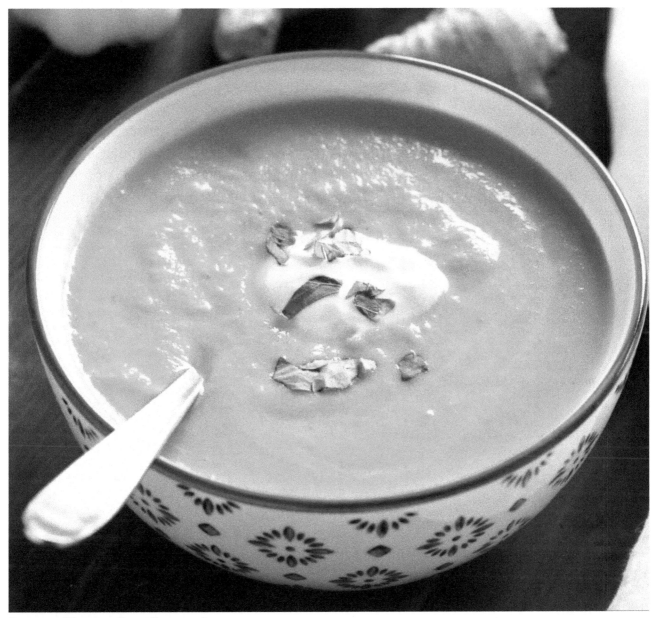

Ingredients for 6 servings:
2 tbsp extra-virgin olive oil 2 onions chopped 1 tsp table salt 1 tbsp grated fresh ginger 1 tbsp ground coriander 1 tbsp ground fennel 1 tsp ground cinnamon 4 cups vegetable or chicken broth 2 cups Water 2 lbs carrots peeled and cut into 2 inch pieces ½ tsp baking soda 2 tbsp pomegranate molasses ½ cup plain greek yogurt ½ cup hazelnuts toasted, skinned, and chopped ½ cup chopped fresh cilantro or mint
Directions and total time – 30-60 m

• Using highest Sauté function, heat oil in Instant Pot until shimmering. Add onions and salt and cook until onions are ¬softened, about 5 minutes. Stir in ginger, coriander, fennel, and cinnamon and cook until fragrant, about 30 seconds. Stir in broth, water, carrots, and baking soda. • Lock lid in place and close pressure release valve. Select Pressure Cook function and cook for 3 minutes. Turn off Instant Pot and quick-release pressure. Carefully remove lid, allowing steam to escape away from you. • Working in batches, process soup in blender until smooth, 1 to 2 minutes. Return processed soup to Instant Pot and bring to simmer using highest Sauté function. Season with salt and pepper to taste. Drizzle individual portions with pomegranate molasses and top with yogurt, hazelnuts, and cilantro before serving.

Bell Peppers Classic
Ingredients for 4 servings:
4 large bell peppers tops removed, seeded and membranes removed 1 cup Cooked rice ½ lb ground beef preferably 93% lean, uncooked 1 egg beaten ¼ cup bread crumbs 2 tbsp tomato paste 4 tsp Worcestershire sauce 1 tbsp chopped parsley additional for garnish 2 tsp Italian seasoning 1 tsp garlic powder 1 tsp onion powder ½ cup marinara sauce

Directions and total time – 15-30 m
• Poke 2 small holes in the bottom of each pepper with a thin knife or toothpick. Set aside. • In a large bowl, combine all remaining ingredients except marinara sauce. • Mound rice mixture into peppers. Do not pack tightly. Mixture should be slightly higher than top of pepper. • Pour one cup of water in the Instant Pot and insert the steam rack. • Place peppers onto rack and divide marinara sauce in the top center of each pepper. • Secure the lid, making sure the vent is closed. • Using the display panel select the MANUAL function. Use the +/- keys and program the Instant Pot for 9 minutes. • When the time is up, quick-release the pressure. Use a meat thermometer to ensure internal temperature is at least 160°F degrees. • (Optional) Place peppers under the broiler for 3-5 minutes to crisp the tops. • Carefully remove the peppers, garnish with additional chopped parsley and serve warm.

Red Curry Cauliflower
Ingredients for 4-6 servings:
14 oz full fat coconut milk 1 can ½ - 1 cup Water 2 tbsp red curry paste 1 tsp garlic powder 1 tsp salt plus more as needed ½ tsp ground ginger ½ tsp onion powder ¼ tsp chili powder (or cayenne pepper) 1 bell pepper any color, thinly sliced 3 - 4 cups cauliflower cut into bite-size pieces (1 small to medium head) 14 oz can diced tomatoes and liquid 1 can freshly ground black pepper Cooked rice or other grain for serving (optional)

Directions and total time – 15-30 m
• In your Instant Pot, stir together the coconut milk, water, red curry paste, garlic powder, salt, ginger, onion powder, and chili powder. Add the bell pepper, cauliflower, and tomatoes, and stir again. Lock the lid and turn the steam release handle to Sealing. Using the Manual or Pressure Cook function, set the cooker to High Pressure for 2 minutes. • When the cook time is complete, quick release the pressure. • Carefully remove the lid and give the whole thing a good stir. Taste and season with more salt and pepper, as needed. Serve with rice or another grain (if using).

Best Creamy Soup
Ingredients for 6 servings:
1 tbsp vegetable oil 1 large Red Bell Pepper diced (about 1 cup) 1 cup frozen whole kernel corn thawed 1 tbsp chili powder 12 oz boneless, skinless chicken breast (2 small or 1 large cut in half lengthwise) 2 cans white cannellini beans about 15 oz each, rinsed and drained 1 cup Salsa 1 cup Water 1 can Condensed Cream of Chicken Soup 10 ½ ounces 5 tbsp shredded Cheddar cheese 2 green onions sliced (about ¼ cup)
Directions and total time – 30-60 m
• On a 6 quart Instant Pot, select the Saute setting. Heat the oil in the Instant Pot. Add the pepper, corn and chili powder and cook for 2 minutes, stirring occasionally. Press Cancel. • Season the chicken with salt and pepper. Layer the beans, salsa, water, chicken and soup over the corn mixture (the order is important, so don't stir until after the cooking is done). Lock the lid and close the pressure release valve. Pressure cook on High pressure, setting the timer to 4 minutes (timer will begin counting down once pressure is reached- it takes about 18 minutes). When done, press Cancel and use the quick release method to release the pressure. • Remove the chicken from the pot. Shred the chicken and return to the pot. Season to taste and serve topped with the cheese and green onions.

Beef Stew Soup
Ingredients for 4 servings:
1 large onion chopped 3 cloves garlic minced 1 ½ cup beef or chicken broth 2 tbsp soy sauce 1 tbsp brown sugar 1 tbsp vinegar any kind 1 tsp salt ½ tsp pepper 1 - 1.5 lbs stew beef frozen or fresh 3 - 4 red-skinned potatoes cut into 1 inch pieces 2 to 3 carrots cut into 1 inch pieces 1 cup frozen peas 2 tbsp cornstarch 3 tbsp Water 2 tbsp chopped fresh parsley optional

Directions and total time – 30-60 m

• Toss the first ten ingredients, up to and including the frozen stew beef, into the Instant Pot. Close the lid and make sure the valve is set to Sealing. Push Pressure Cook (or Manual) and use the +/– button to get to 25 minutes. • While it's cooking, cut the potatoes and carrots into 1" pieces, with or without the skins. Make a slurry by stirring the cornstarch into the water until smooth. • When the pot beeps that it's done, leave it for a 10-minute natural release. Then flip the valve to Venting for a quick release of any remaining pressure and when the pin drops, open the pot. • Toss in the potatoes and carrots (not the peas) and gently push them into the liquid. Close the lid again and hit Pressure Cook (or Manual). Set the cook time to 4 minutes. When it's done, do a quick release - pin drop - open the pot. • Hit Cancel, then Saute. Give the cornstarch slurry a stir and when the stew is boiling stir in about half the slurry. Boil to thicken it and if you want it thicker, add more of the slurry. • Hit Cancel and stir in the frozen peas. The heat of the stew will be enough to cook them without turning them to mush. Taste and add salt and pepper if needed. Add the parsley, if using, and You. Are. Done. • Go back to bed. And I hope you feel better soon.

Greek Salad with Bulgur Wheat
Ingredients for 2 servings:

½ cup coarse bulgur wheat ½ cup Water ¼ tsp kosher salt ⅓ cup English cucumber chopped ½ cup fresh tomatoes chopped 1 scallion green part only, sliced 2 tbsp Kalamata olives coarsely chopped ¼ cup extra-virgin olive oil 2 tbsp lemon juice freshly squeezed ⅓ cup feta cheese crumbled 1 tbsp fresh mint chopped ¼ cup fresh parsley chopped

Directions and total time – 15 m

• Pour the bulgur into the inner pot. Add the water and kosher salt. Lock the lid into place. Select Pressure Cook or Manual, and adjust the pressure to High and the time to 0 minutes. After cooking, let the pressure release naturally for 2 minutes, then quick release any remaining pressure. • Unlock the lid. Remove the pot from the base. Fluff the bulgur with a fork and let it cool for a few minutes. Transfer it to a medium bowl. • Add the cucumber, tomatoes, scallion, and olives, and toss to combine. Drizzle with the olive oil and lemon juice. Add the feta cheese, mint, and parsley, and toss gently. Adjust the seasoning, adding salt or pepper as needed.

Cheesy Vegetable Strata

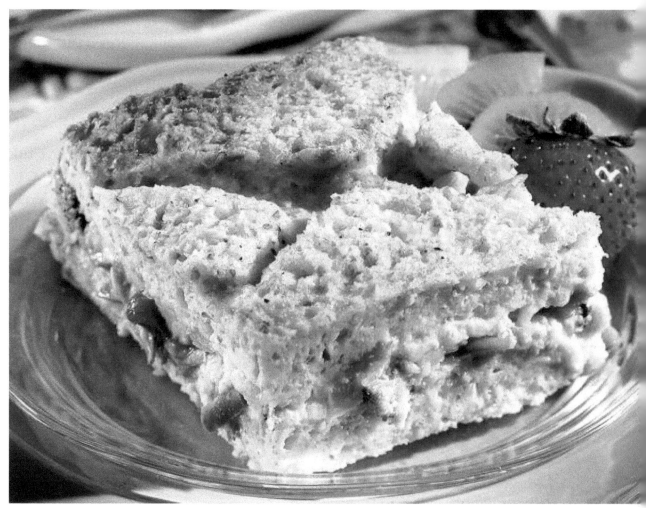

Ingredients for 4 servings:

Dry ingredients: ¼ cup dried Parmesan cheese 2 tbsp dried yellow or green onion ¼ cup dried green bell pepper 2 tbsp sundried tomatoes 1 tbsp dried parsley 1 tsp sea salt ½ tsp ground black pepper 4 cups dry cubed bread For cooking and serving: Cooking Spray 8 eggs ½ cup heavy cream 1 cup Water

Directions and total time – 15-30 m

• Layer the dry ingredients in the jar in the order listed. To Cook: • Coat the bottom and sides of a 7 cup Pyrex dish or fluted tube pan, such as a Bundt pan, with cooking spray. Place all of the jarred ingredients into the baking dish. In a separate jar, whisk the eggs and heavy cream. Pour this mixture into the pan, press down on the bread to submerge it beneath the egg mixture, and stir gently to disperse the ingredients. Cover the pan with aluminum foil. Pour 1 cup of water into the Instant Pot and place the trivet into the pot. Use a foil sling (if needed) to place the baking dish on top of the trivet. Cover the Instant Pot with the lid and ensure the vent is in the "Sealed" position. Pressure Cook on High for 20 minutes. Allow the steam pressure to release naturally for 10 minutes, then release any remaining pressure manually.

Savory Barbacoa Beef
Ingredients for 6-8 servings:

Marinade Mixture: 6 oz beer or water 4 oz diced green chiles 1 can 1 small onion finely diced 4 cloves garlic 3 in chipotlesadobo sauce or to taste ¼ cup lime juice 2 tbsp apple cider vinegar 1 tbsp cumin 2 tsp dried oregano leaves 1 tsp pepper ¼ tsp ground cloves Savory Barbacoa Beef: 1 tbsp olive oil 3 lb lbs beef chuck roast (if more than 2 inch thick, cut into 1chunks) 3 bay leaves 1 tbsp kosher salt or to taste For Serving: tortillas Diced avocado chopped cilantro diced red onion Lime wedges

Directions and total time – 1-2 h

• Combine Marinade Mixture ingredients in a blender and process until completely smooth. • Add olive oil to the Instant Pot. Using the display panel select the SAUTE function. • When oil gets hot, brown the meat on both sides, 3-4 minutes per side. Meat will not be cooked through. • Add marinade to the pot and deglaze by using a wooden spoon to scrape the brown bits from the bottom of the pot. • Add bay leaves, then toss to ensure everything is coated in the marinade. • Turn the pot off by selecting CANCEL, then secure the lid, making sure the vent is closed. • Using the display panel select the MANUAL or PRESSURE COOK function. Use the +/- keys and program the Instant Pot for 60 minutes. • When the time is up, let the pressure naturally release for 15 minutes, then quick-release the remaining pressure. • Discard bay leaves. Carefully remove the meat from the pot to a cutting board and shred. • (Optional) Skim fat off the top of the sauce using a large spoon or gravy separator. • Return the meat to the pot, add salt and toss to coat. • Serve shredded beef in tacos, salads, burrito bowls, or nachos alongside lime wedges.

Potato Corn Chowder
Ingredients for 6 servings:
4 slices bacon diced 3 cloves garlic minced 1 onion finely diced 4 cups chicken broth warmed 1 ½ lbs red potatoes unpeeled, cut into a 1 inch dice 16 oz frozen corn kernels 2 tsp sprigs fresh thyme or 1 dried thyme ¾ cup heavy cream 3 tbsp flour Pinch of cayenne salt and pepper to taste 2 tbsp snipped fresh chives for garnish optional

Directions and total time – 15-30 m
• Add bacon to the Instant Pot. Using the display panel select the SAUTÉ function and adjust to MORE or HIGH. Cook and stir until bacon is crisp. Remove bacon to a paper towel-lined plate, reserving drippings. • Add onion to the drippings and Sauté until it begins to soften, 2-3 minutes. Add garlic and cook for 1-2 minutes more. • Add warmed broth to the pot and deglaze by using a wooden spoon to scrape the brown bits from the bottom of the pot. • Add potatoes, corn and thyme sprigs to the pot and stir, then secure the lid, making sure the vent is closed. • Using the display panel select the MANUAL or PRESSURE COOK function. Use the +/- keys and program the Instant Pot for 10 minutes. • When the time is up, quick-release the remaining pressure. • Remove the thyme sprigs and discard. Return the pot to SAUTÉ mode and bring to a boil. • In a small bowl, whisk together cream, flour and cayenne. Add to boiling pot and cook and stir until slightly thickened, 4-5 minutes. Add salt and pepper to taste. • Serve immediately, garnished with bacon and (optional) chives. • scallions, if desired

Lasagna in Mug
Ingredients for 1 servings:
2 tbsp whole milk ricotta cheese 2 tbsp full-fat Cheddar cheese shredded ½ cup full-fat Parmesan cheese grated ½ Zucchini thinly sliced tsp basil dried ½ tsp oregano dried ½ tsp freshly ground black pepper ½ tsp kosher salt ½ cup full-fat mozzarella cheese shredded 6 oz sugar-free or low-sugar roasted tomatoes ½ can drained

Directions and total time – 15 m
• Pour 1 cup filtered water into the Instant Pot, then insert the trivet. In a large bowl, combine the ricotta, Cheddar, Parmesan, zucchini, basil, oregano, black pepper, salt, mozzarella, and tomatoes. Mix thoroughly. Transfer this mixture into a well-greased, Instant Pot–friendly mug (or multiple, smaller mugs, if desired). • Place the mug onto the trivet, and cover loosely with aluminum foil. Close the lid, set the pressure release to Sealing, and select Manual/Pressure Cook. Set the Instant Pot to 5 minutes on high pressure and let cook. • Once cooked, let the pressure naturally disperse from the Instant Pot for about 10 minutes, then carefully switch the pressure release to Venting. • Open the Instant Pot, and remove the mug. Let cool, serve, and enjoy!

Spinach Spaghetti with Sausage
Ingredients for 4 servings:
1 lb italian sausage sliced 1 box frozen spinach thawed and squeezed of all liquids ½ onion diced 24 oz spaghetti sauce 8 oz spaghetti broken in half 1 tsp Italian seasoning generous tsp 1 tsp garlic powder Salt and pepper as desired 3 cup chicken broth or water 1 tbsp oil

Directions and total time – 15-30 m
• In the Instant Pot inner pot, place the sausage, onions, Italian seasoning, garlic powder, salt and pepper and and press SAUTE on the IP. • Saute the mixture until it's cooked through and the onions are tender. • Add the spaghetti sauce, water/broth, and dry spaghetti noodles. • Mix every well (make sure all noodles are covered in liquid) and place the lid on the Instant Pot, and bringing the toggle switch into the "seal" position. • Press MANUAL or PRESSURE COOK and adjust time for 5 minutes. • When the five minutes are up, do a natural release for 5 minutes and then move the toggle switch to "Vent" to release the rest of the pressure in the pot. • Remove the lid. If the mixture looks watery, press "Saute", and bring the mixture up to a boil and let it boil for a few minutes. It will thicken as it boils. Add the spinach to the pot, stir and let warm through for a few minutes. • Serve and garnish with garlic toast.

Barley Lunch Jars
Ingredients for 5 servings:

1 cup pearl barley ½ teaspoon salt 4 cups water 2 ½ cups salad greens 10 to 12 cherry tomatoes, halved 5 small sweet peppers, sliced 2 small cucumbers, sliced 5 radishes, sliced Vinaigrette, for serving Special equipment: 6-quart Instant Pot or other pressure cooker 5 pint jars, for assembly

Directions and total time – 30-60 m

• Add dried barley to your Instant Pot or other multi cooker/pressure cooker. Stir in salt and water. Replace lid and cook on high pressure for 15 minutes. • Once finished, let pressure naturally release for five minutes. Vent steam, remove lid, drain off any extra water, and let barley cool to room temperature. • Instant Pot Barley Lunch Jars - barley in water in pressure cooker. How to cook Barley grains of barley in hand. • There's no single way to assemble these lunch jars. I like to add ½ cup of cooked barley to the bottom (make sure it is room temperature). Top that with a mix of salad greens and lots of sliced vegetables. • Is Barley Gluten-Free? jar with barley in bottomInstant Pot Barley Lunch Jars - jars stuffed with vegetables • The jars will keep in the fridge for 4-5 days. After that the greens start to wilt. You cannot freeze these jars. They are intended to be made and eaten within the week. • When it's time for lunch, drizzle vinaigrette into the jar, season with a pinch of salt and pepper, then eat the barley salad right out of the jar. Alternatively, pour onto a plate. (Don't add the vinaigrette to the salad until right before serving, as it will make the vegetables soggy.).

Healthy Chicken Soup

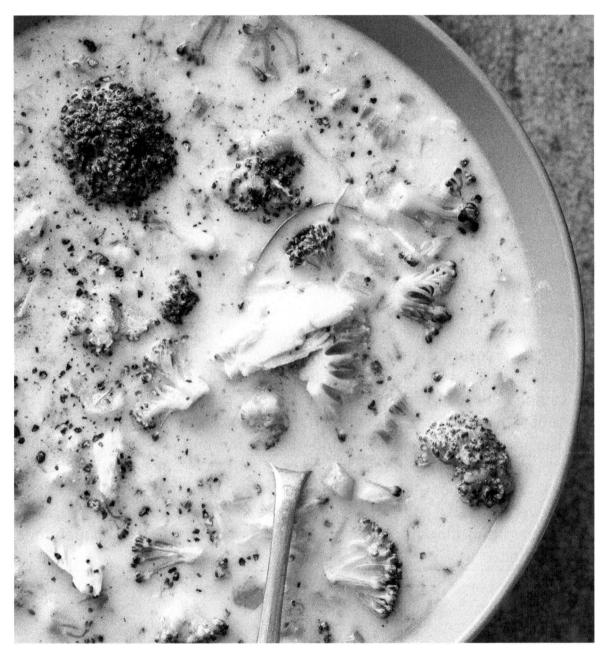

Ingredients for 4-6 servings:
1 3- to 4-pound chicken, or an equivalent mix of bone-in thighs, legs, or breast meat 4 ribs celery, sliced 3 medium carrots, peeled and sliced 1 medium parsnip, halved lengthwise and sliced 1 medium yellow onion, diced 3 cloves garlic, smashed and peeled 12 sprigs fresh flat leaf parsley 3 large sprigs fresh thyme 4 teaspoons salt 2 quarts water Cooked egg noodles, optional

Directions and total time – 15-30 m

• Put the chicken in the pot of a pressure cooker, breast side up. • Layer all of the other ingredients into the pot, pouring in the water last to avoid splashing. Adding four teaspoons of salt at this point will result in a well-seasoned soup broth. Use less salt or eliminate if you'd like to make basic chicken broth to use for other purposes. • Cook the soup: Place the lid on the pressure cooker. Make sure the pressure regulator is set to the "Sealing" position. Select the "Manual" program, then set the time to 25 minutes at high pressure. (Instant Pot users can also select the "Soup" program and follow the same cooking time. For stovetop pressure cookers, cook at high pressure for 22 minutes.) It will take about 35 minutes for your pressure cooker to come up to pressure, and then the actual cooking will begin. Total time from the time you seal the pressure cooker to the finished dish is about one hour. • When the soup has finished cooking, wait about 15 minutes before "quick" releasing the pressure. This helps prevent a lot of steamy broth spitting out of the valve. Even so be careful when releasing the steam! You can also let the pressure release naturally, though this will take quite a while. Wait until the pressure cooker's float valve has returned to its "down" position before opening the pressure cooker. • Prepare the chicken meat: Use a pair of tongs or a slotted spoon to remove the chicken from the pot, and transfer it to a dish to cool until you can comfortably handle it, about 20 minutes. It may come apart as you are removing it from the pot, so go slowly and carefully. Take the meat off of the bones, and discard the bones, skin, and cartilage. Cut or tear the meat into bite-sized pieces. • Stir the chicken meat back into the soup. Ladle into bowls and serve. Add cooked egg noodles, if you like. Let any leftover soup cool completely, then store in the fridge for up to 5 days or freeze for up to 3 months. The soup may gel as it cools; it will liquefy again when heated.

Mashed Potatoes
Ingredients for 6-8 servings:
1 cup water 3 to 3 ½ pounds (4 large) russet potatoes, peeled and sliced 1-inch thick 4 cloves garlic, peeled (optional) ¾ cup whole milk 3 tablespoons unsalted butter 1 ½ teaspoons kosher salt
½ teaspoon freshly ground black pepper Chopped fresh chives or parsley, for garnish (optional)

Directions and total time – 15-30 m
• Pressure cook the potatoes and garlic: Place a steamer basket in the bottom of your electric pressure cooker and add 1 cup of water. Add the sliced potatoes and peeled garlic cloves (if using) on top of the steamer basket. Secure the lid on your pressure cooker and make sure the pressure release valve is set to its "sealing" position. Select the "Steam" or "Manual" setting and set the cooking time to 4 minutes at high pressure. (The pot will take about 15 minutes to come up to pressure and then the actual cooking will begin). When the cooking program ends, perform a quick release by moving the pressure release valve to its "venting" position. • Drain the water from the pot, then put the potatoes and garlic back in: Use heatproof mitts to remove the steamer basket from the pot. Lift out the inner pot and pour out the water, then return the potatoes to the inner pot of the pressure cooker (don't put it back in the pressure cooker housing). • Mash the potatoes, then taste for seasoning: Add the milk, butter, salt, and pepper. Use a potato masher to work the ingredients into the potatoes, mashing until the potatoes are mashed as much as you like them. Add more milk or butter if you like. Taste the potatoes for seasoning, and add more salt and/or pepper if needed. • Spoon the potatoes into a serving bowl and sprinkle the chopped chives on top. Serve hot.

Green Beans with Tomatoes and Bacon
Ingredients for 4-6 servings:
4 slices thick-sliced bacon (about 4 ounces), cut into 1-inch pieces 1 medium onion, diced 1 pound green beans, stem ends trimmed 1 (14.5-ounce) can diced tomatoes ⅓ cup water ¼ teaspoon salt ¼ teaspoon ground black pepper ⅛ teaspoon cayenne pepper 2 sprigs fresh thyme

Directions and total time – 30-60 m
• Cook the bacon and onions in the pressure cooker: Select the "Sauté" setting and add the bacon to the pressure cooker. (If you are using a stovetop pressure cooker, use medium heat.). Let the bacon cook until it has rendered some fat and begun to brown a bit, about 7 minutes. Add the onions and sauté until softened and translucent, about 3 more minutes. • Stir in the rest of the ingredients and pressure cook: Add the green beans, diced tomatoes and their liquid, water, salt, pepper, cayenne, and thyme. Give everything a good stir so all of the green beans are coated with some of the cooking liquid. Secure the lid on the pressure cooker. Make sure that the pressure regulator is set to the "Sealing" position. Cancel the "Sauté" program on the pressure cooker, then select the "Manual" or "Pressure Cook" setting. Set the cooking time to 7 minutes at high pressure. (For stovetop pressure cookers, cook for 6 minutes at high pressure.). It will take about 10 minutes for your pressure cooker to come up to pressure, and then the 7 minutes of actual cooking will begin. • Release the pressure: Perform a quick pressure release by immediately moving the vent from "Sealing" to "Venting" (be careful of the steam!). The pot will take a couple minutes to fully release the pressure. • Serve the green beans: Use a slotted spoon to gently transfer the green beans to a serving dish. Scoop up the tomatoes, bacon, and onions, and spoon them over the top of the beans. Serve hot.

Mushroom Risotto
Ingredients for 4-6 servings:
2 tablespoons extra virgin olive oil 1 pound mushrooms, washed, trimmed, and quartered or sliced 1 medium onion, finely diced 3 cloves garlic, minced ¼ teaspoon salt or to taste ¼ teaspoon freshly ground black pepper or to taste 2 cups Arborio or Carnaroli rice ½ cup dry white wine 2 teaspoons soy sauce 2 teaspoons miso paste (white or red) 3 ¾ to 4 cups low-sodium chicken or vegetable stock, divided 2 tablespoons unsalted butter ½ cup finely shredded parmesan cheese, plus more to garnish ¼ teaspoon lemon zest, optional

Directions and total time – 30-60 m
• Sauté the mushrooms: Select "Sauté" on the Instant Pot and adjust the heat to high. Add the oil to the cooker. When the oil shimmers, add the mushrooms and cook, stirring occasionally, until the liquid evaporates and the mushrooms are slightly browned, about 15 minutes. (If it seems like a long time, it's because it is. Liquid takes longer to evaporate in the deep pot of the pressure cooker.) • Sauté the onions and garlic: Once the mushrooms are fully cooked, add the onions and garlic to the Instant Pot and cook until the onion is translucent, about 3 minutes. Sprinkle with salt and pepper to taste. • Add the rice: Add the rice and cook, stirring, until the grains are coated in the oil and the outer parts of the rice kernels are translucent, 1-2 minutes. Add the wine and cook, stirring, until nearly all the wine is evaporated, about 3 minutes. (This keeps the wine from having a raw taste, which can happen in a pressure cooker.) • Season and cook under pressure: Stir in the soy sauce, miso, and 3 ¾ cup stock. Secure the lid, and make sure the pressure release valve is set to seal. Program the Instant Pot to cook on Manual/Pressure at high pressure for 5 minutes. (It will take about 10 minutes for the Instant Pot to come to pressure.). When the Instant Pot beeps, release the pressure using the quick release: depending on the model of cooker you have, you will do this by pushing a button on the pressure cooker or nudge the valve open with the handle of a long spoon to keep your fingers away from the steam. Unlock the lid and open it. There will be a layer of thick liquid at the top of the pot and the rice will mostly be at the bottom. Stir to combine. • Check for doneness: Carefully taste a bit of the risotto. You are checking for doneness— you want the rice to have a little bite, but not be raw and crunchy. If it's loose and soupy or if it's crunchy, turn on the "Sauté" setting and cook with the lid off. If loose stir constantly, until more of the liquid has been absorbed by the rice. If it's crunchy add the remaining ¼ cup stock and stir until it's absorbed

a bit, about 1 minute. You want the consistency to be "all'onda" ("like waves" in Italian). It's the risottoland happy place between soupy/watery and gloppy/stiff. You want it to be rich and creamy. • Finish the risotto: Stir in the butter and parmesan. Taste one more time for seasoning. If it seems a little too earthy and flat, add the ¼ teaspoon of lemon zest. Adjust with salt, if needed. Serve right away.

Cube-Steak and Gravy
Ingredients for 4 servings:
1-2 pounds cube steak 1 10 oz can french onion soup 1 packet of Au Jus Gravy Mix 10 oz water 1 tbs steak sauce optional 2 tbs corn starch

Directions and total time – 15-30 m
• Place steak in your IP Pour over gravy mix • Pour in your can of onion soup and fill the same can with water and pour in. • Place your IP on Manual High Pressure for 4 minutes. • Do a natural release for 5 minutes then quick release and place your instant pot on saute. • Bring to a boil and whisk in cornstarch if your gravy is not thick enough. • Serve and enjoy!

Shrimp Scampi
Ingredients for 2-4 servings:
1lb shrimp de-veined and peeled, leave tail on ½ Lemon 2 tbls butter whatever you use 3 garlic cloves minced ¼ cup dry white wine used for flavor ½ cup chicken broth dried parsley kosher salt fresh ground pepper

Directions and total time – 30-60 m
• Put pot on saute mode. • When Hot put in butter, let it melt. • Then Saute the garlic till brown. • Add the wine and Saute till the alcohol smell goes away. Use whatever white wine you like. When the alcohol boils away, it leaves an almost sweet taste and the flavor comes from the wine.. • Put in shrimp with the chicken broth, 2 pinches of kosher salt, pepper to taste. • Close the lid and seal it. • Cook on Manual/ High Pressure for 1 min. (if frozen, 3 mins) • Quick release. • Saute again till sauce starts to simmer, • then add ½ Lemon juice and the parsley. Use as much parsley as you want, mix it together and you're done.

Modern Moroccan Chicken Wraps

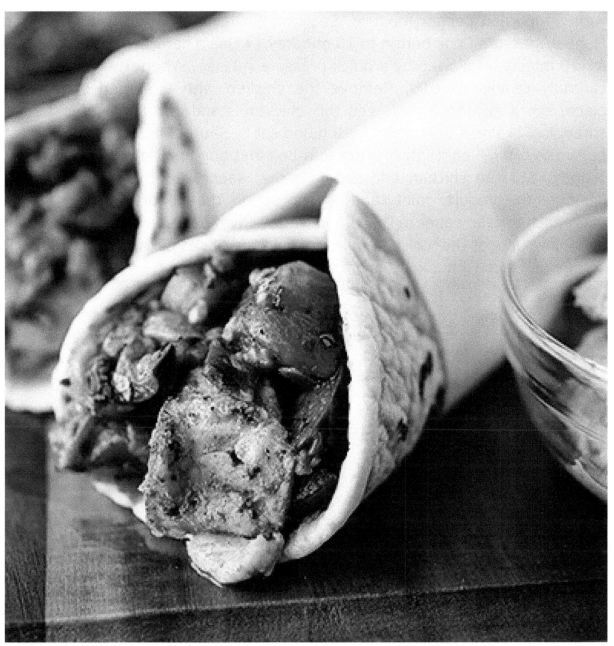

Ingredients for 6 servings:

1 cup roasted red peppers drained 1 tsp ground coriander 1 tsp ground cumin 1 tsp garlic powder ½ tsp ground chipotle pepper ½ tsp caraway seeds ½ cup Water 1 lb boneless skinless chicken thighs trimmed of fat ¼ tsp salt ¾ cup plain 2% Greek yogurt ½ cup chopped fresh mint ⅓ cup finely chopped red onion 6 light flour tortillas heated in a skillet until slightly charred 1 lemon cut into 6 wedges

Directions and total time – 30-60 m • Combine the peppers, coriander, cumin, garlic powder, chipotle, caraway, and water in a blender. Secure the lid and purée until smooth. • Place the chicken thighs in the Instant Pot. Top with the puréed pepper mixture. Seal the lid, close the valve, and set the Manual/Pressure Cook button to 10 minutes. • Use a natural pressure release for 10 minutes, followed by a quick pressure release. When the valve drops, carefully remove the lid. Remove the chicken with a slotted spoon and place on a cutting board. Let the chicken stand for 5 minutes before shredding. • Press the Cancel button and set to Sauté. Then press the Adjust button to "More" or "High." Bring to a boil and boil for 5 minutes to thicken slightly. Stir the chicken and salt into the sauce. • In a medium bowl, combine the yogurt, mint, and onion. Spoon the yogurt mixture evenly over each tortilla, squeeze the lemon wedges over each serving, and top with equal amounts of the chicken mixture. Fold the edges of the tortillas over or serve open face with a knife and fork, if desired.

Black-Eyed Peas
Ingredients for 6-8 servings:
¼ cup real bacon bits 2 tablespoons smoked paprika ¼ teaspoon red chile flakes ⅓ cup dried onion 2 teaspoons dried garlic ¼ cup dried celery ¼ cup dried bell pepper 1 teaspoon dried thyme 1 teaspoon sea salt 2 ¾ cups dried black-eyed peas 6 cups chicken broth or water 1 tablespoon balsamic vinegar to serve

Directions and total time – 30-60 m • Layer the dry ingredients in the jar in the order listed. • Place all of the jarred ingredients into the Instant Pot. Add 6 cups of chicken broth or water. Stir to mix. Cover with the lid and ensure the vent is in the "Sealed" position. Pressure Cook or Manualon High for 20 minutes. Allow the steam pressure to release naturally for 15 minutes, then release any remaining pressure manually.

Tacos: Sweet Potato and Black Bean
Ingredients for 4-6 servings:

1 tablespoons to olive oil ½ sweet onion diced 1 large sweet potato diced 1 red bell pepper diced 1 garlic clove minced 1 tomato diced 15 ounce black beans 1 can rinsed and drained, 1 in canned chipotle pepperadobo sauce diced 1 teaspoons to 2adobo sauce from the can 1 teaspoons to 2chili powder ½ teaspoon salt ½ teaspoon ground cumin ½ cup DIY Vegetable Stock or store-bought stock 1 tablespoon freshly squeezed lime juice 1 lime zested Corn or flour tortillas for serving 1 avocado peeled, pitted, and mashed ¼ cup fresh cilantro chopped Cashew Sour Cream for serving (optional) Garden Salsa for serving (optional), Sliced jalapeño peppers for serving (optional) Sliced red cabbage for serving (optional)

Directions and total time – 15-30 m

• On your Instant Pot, select Sauté Low. When the display reads "Hot," add the oil and heat until it shimmers. Add the onion. Cook for 1 minute, stirring. Add the sweet potato and bell pepper. Cook for 1 minute, stirring so nothing burns. Turn off the Instant Pot and add the garlic. Cook for 30 seconds to 1 minute, stirring. • Add the tomato, black beans, chipotle, adobo sauce, chili powder, salt, cumin, stock, and lime juice. Lock the lid and turn the steam release handle to Sealing. Using the Manual function, set the cooker to High Pressure for 4 minutes (3 minutes at sea level). • When the cook time is complete, turn off the Instant Pot and let the pressure release naturally for 5 minutes; quick release any remaining pressure. • Carefully remove the lid. If there is too much liquid in the inner pot, select Sauté Low again and cook for 1 to 2 minutes, stirring constantly (it gets hot fast!). • Stir in the lime zest. Serve in the tortillas, topped with mashed avocado and cilantro and anything else your heart desires. Warm

Buffalo Cauliflower Bites
 Ingredients for 4 servings:
1 head cauliflower (large) cut into large pieces ½ cup buffalo hot sauce
Directions and total time – 15 m
• Pour 1 cup water into the Instant Pot and place the steam rack inside. •
Place the cauliflower in a 7-cup glass bowl and add the buffalo hot sauce. Toss
to evenly coat. Place the bowl on top of the steam rack. Secure the lid. •
Press the Manual or Pressure Cook button and adjust the time to 2 minutes. •
When the timer beeps, quick-release pressure until float valve drops and then
unlock lid. • Transfer to a plate and serve with toothpicks.

Mac, Cheese & Meatballs
Ingredients for 4 servings:

4 cups chicken or vegetable broth 1 quart 1 lb mini or bite-sized frozen turkey meatballs (even vegan and/or gluten-free meatballs, if that's a concern), ½-1 ounce each 4 tbsp butter ½ stick 2 tsp stemmed fresh thyme leaves or 1 teaspoon dried thyme 1 tsp onion powder 1 tsp garlic powder ½ tsp table salt 16 ounce elbow macaroni or gluten-free elbow macaroni, not "giant" or "jumbo" macaroni 12 ounces shredded cheddar Swiss, mozzarella, Havarti, Monterey Jack, or other semi-firm cheese, or even a blend of cheeses (3 cups) 1 ounce finely grated Parmigiano-Reggiano ½ cup ½ cup heavy cream or light cream, but not "fat-free"½ cup marinara sauce

Directions and total time – 30-60 m

• Press the button SAUTÉ. Set it for HIGH, MORE, or CUSTOM 400°F and set the timer for 10 minutes. • Mix the broth, meatballs, butter, thyme, onion powder, garlic powder, and salt in an Instant Pot. Heat until many wisps of steam rise from the liquid. Turn off the SAUTÉ function. Stir in the macaroni and lock the lid onto the pot. • Option 1 Max Pressure Cooker Press Pressure cook on Max pressure for 5 minutes with the Keep Warm setting off. • Option 2 All Pressure Cookers Press Meat/Stew or Pressure cook (Manual) on High pressure for 6 minutes with the Keep Warm setting off. The valve must be closed. • Use the quick-release method to bring the pot's pressure back to normal. Unlatch the lid and open the cooker. • Press the button SAUTÉ. Set it for HIGH, MORE, or CUSTOM 400°F and set the timer for 5 minutes. • Stir in the shredded cheese, grated Parmesan, and cream until the cheese is melted and bubbly. Turn off the SAUTÉ function; set the lid askew over the pot and let sit for a couple of minutes. Serve warm.

Tater Tot Soup
Ingredients for 6-8 servings:
6 cups chicken or vegetable broth 1 ½ quarts 2 tbsp butter 2 tsp peeled and minced garlic 2 tsp dried basil oregano, or thyme 1 tsp onion powder ½ tsp ground black pepper 1 lb frozen unseasoned hash brown cubes (3 cups, NOT frozen shredded hash browns) 5 cups frozen Tater Tots or potato puffs; 1 ¼ lbs 2 cups shredded mild or sharp Cheddar cheese; 8 ounces

Directions and total time – 15-30 m
• Press the button SAUTÉ. Set it for HIGH, MORE, or CUSTOM 400°F and set the time for 10 minutes. • Mix the broth, butter, garlic, dried herb, onion powder, and pepper in an Instant Pot. Heat, stirring occasionally, until wisps of steam rise from the liquid. Stir in the hash brown cubes and Tater Tots. Lock the lid onto the pot. • Option 1 Max Pressure Cooker Press Pressure cook on Max pressure for 3 minutes with the Keep Warm setting off. • Option 2 All Pressure Cookers Press SOUP/BROIL or Pressure Cook (Manual) on High pressure for 4 minutes with the Keep Warm setting off. The valve must be closed. • Use the quick-release method to bring the pot's pressure back to normal. Unlatch the lid and open the cooker. Stir in the cheese. Set the lid askew over the pot for a couple of minutes until the cheese melts. Stir again, then serve hot.

Bone-In Chicken Breasts

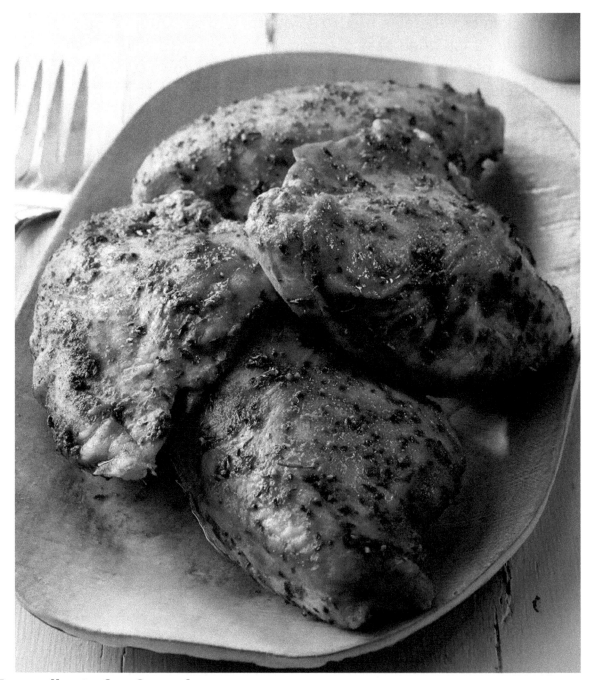

Ingredients for 6 servings:
1 cup liquid. Choose from water, broth of any sort, wine of any sort, beer of any sort, unsweetened apple cider or a combination of any of these. 6 frozen bone-in skin-on chicken breasts 12-14 ounces 2 tbsp dried seasoning blend. Choose from Provençal, Cajun, poultry, taco, Italian, or another blend you prefer or create. 1 ½ tsp table salt. Optional
Directions and total time – 30-60 m

• Pour the liquid into an Instant Pot. Position the bone-in chicken breasts in the liquid in a crisscross pattern (rather than stacking them on top of each other) so that steam can circulate among them. Sprinkle the top of each with 1 tsp dried seasoning blend and ¼ tsp salt (if using). Lock the lid onto the pot. • Optional 1 Max Pressure Cooker Press Pressure cook on Max pressure for 35 minutes with the Keep Warm setting off. • Optional 2 All Pressure Cookers Press Poultry, Pressure Cook or Manual on High pressure for 40 minutes with the Keep Warm setting off. (The Valve must be closed) • Use the quick-release method to bring the pot's pressure back to normal. Unlatch the lid and open the cooker. Insert an instant-read meat thermometer into the center of a couple of the breasts, without touching bone, to make sure their internal temperature is 165°F. The meat can be a little pink at the bone and still perfectly safe to eat, so long as its internal temperature is correct. If the internal temperature is below 165°F (or if you're worried about the color), lock the lid back onto the pot and give the breasts 3 extra minutes at MAX, or 4 minutes at HIGH. Again, use the quick-release method to bring the pot's pressure back to normal. • Use kitchen tongs to transfer the breasts to serving plates or a serving platter to serve. Or cool them at room temperature for 10 minutes or so, then store in a sealed container in the fridge for up to 3 days.

Kabocha Squash Soup with Lemongrass and Ginger
Ingredients for 4 servings:
1 ½ tbsp grapeseed oil or other neutral high-heat cooking oil 1 Kabocha squash 1 large yellow onion diced 2 medium carrots diced 4 garlic cloves minced 2- inch piece fresh ginger grated or minced 3 Thai green chile peppers thinly sliced (seeded for a milder heat or omit entirely) 4 cups low sodium vegetable broth 2 large Fuji apples unpeeled and roughly chopped 1 ½ tsp kosher salt 13.5 ounce full fat coconut milk 1 can 1 tbsp reduced-sodium tamari or soy sauce 2 pieces lemongrass stalks tough outer layers removed and stalks cut into 6-inch, optional but highly recommended 1 to 2 tsp fresh lime juice to taste

Directions and total time – 15-30 m
• Using a large, sharp knife, halve the squash through the stem and cut off the stem. You may need to microwave the whole squash for 2 to 3 minutes to soften it and make it easier to slice. Once halved, use a large spoon to scoop out the seeds and gunk. Cut each half into 3 or 4 wedges, lay each wedge flat on its side, and use a knife to cut the peel off. Then, cut the squash into 1 ½-inch chunks. You should end up with about 5 cups of squash. • Select the Sauté setting on the Instant Pot and, after a few minutes, add the oil. Once the display reads "HOT," add the onion and carrots and cook for 5 minutes, stirring occasionally, until the onion begins to brown. • Add the garlic, ginger, and chiles (if using) and cook for 1 minute, stirring frequently. • Pour in the vegetable broth to deglaze the pan and use a wooden spoon to scrape up any browned bits on the bottom of the pot. Add the kabocha squash, apples, salt, coconut milk, tamari, and lemongrass. Stir to combine well. Select the Cancel setting. • Secure the lid and set the Pressure Release to Sealing. Select the Soup setting at high pressure and set the cook time to 12 minutes. • Once the 12-minute timer has completed and beeps, allow a natural pressure release for 5 minutes and then switch the Pressure Release knob from Sealing to Venting to release any remaining steam. • Open the pot and discard the lemongrass stalks. Using an immersion blender, puree the soup for a few minutes until you have a thick and creamy soup. (Alternatively, blend the soup in batches in a high-powered blender. Be sure to remove the center cap from the blender lid to vent steam, but cover the hole with a kitchen towel.) • Stir in 1 tsp lime juice and taste. Add another tsp of lime juice, if desired, and adjust the seasonings accordingly. Transfer the soup to bowls and garnish as desired.

Lite Tabasco Mac
Ingredients for 4-6 servings:

1 lbs elbow macaroni 4 cups Water 1 tsp fine sea salt Sauce: 1 cup raw cashews soaked in water for 2 hours at room temperature, or up to overnight in the refrigerator, and drained ⅓ cup Water plus more if needed 2 tbsp nutritional yeast 1 ½ tbsp fresh lemon juice 1 clove garlic peeled 1 tsp prepared yellow mustard 1 tsp Tabasco sauce ½ tsp fine sea salt plus more as needed ¼ tsp cayenne pepper plus more as needed

Directions and total time – 15 m

• Secure the lid and set the Pressure Release to Sealing. Select the Manual or Pressure Cook setting and set the cooking time for 6 minutes at High pressure. (The pot will take about 15 minutes to come up to pressure before the cooking program begins.) • To make the sauce: While the pasta is cooking, combine the cashews, water, nutritional yeast, lemon juice, garlic, mustard, Tabasco, salt, and cayenne in a blender. Blend at high speed for about 1 minute, until smooth, scraping down the sides of the blender halfway through, if necessary. Taste for seasoning, adding more salt and/or cayenne, if needed. You can also add an extra splash of water, if you prefer a thinner sauce. • When the cooking program ends, let the pressure release naturally for 5 minutes, then move the Pressure Release to Venting to release any remaining steam. Open the pot and stir in the sauce. • Spoon the macaroni into bowls and serve immediately.

Creamy Shrimp Bisque
Ingredients for 4 servings:

1 lb peeled and deveined shrimp roughly chopped ½ tsp kosher salt ¼ tsp pepper 1 tbsp butter 1 tbsp olive oil ½ cup diced onion ½ cup diced celery 1 cup diced carrots 3 cloves garlic minced 2 tbsp brandy 1 ½ cups broth warmed 2 lbs tomatoes quartered ½ cup heavy cream 1 tbsp fresh chives snipped

Directions and total time – 15-30 m

• Season the shrimp with salt and pepper, then add butter to the Instant Pot. Using the display panel select the SAUTE function. • When butter melts, add shrimp and cook, tossing occasionally, until opaque throughout, 3 - 4 minutes. Transfer shrimp to a shallow dish and cover loosely with foil. • Add olive oil to the pot. When oil is hot, add onion, celery, and carrots to the pot and saute until softened, 3 - 4 minutes. Add garlic and cook for 1 - 2 minutes more. • Add brandy to the pot and cook for 30 seconds, then add broth to the pot and deglaze by using a wooden spoon to scrape the brown bits from the bottom of the pot. • Add tomatoes to the pot and stir to combine. • Turn the pot off by selecting CANCEL, then secure the lid, making sure the vent is closed. • Using the display panel select the MANUAL or PRESSURE COOK function. Use the +/- keys and program the Instant Pot for 8 minutes. • When the time is up, quick-release the pressure, then use an immersion blender to puree the soup. • Stir in heavy cream, adjust seasonings, then ladle the soup into bowls and top with the shrimp and chives.

Jerk Chicken & Cornbread
Ingredients for 4 servings:
Chicken and Cornbread: 8.5 oz corn muffin mix 1 box, prepared according to package directions 2 tbsp Thinly sliced scallions 1 jalapeno seeded and minced 1 tbsp olive oil ⅓ cup chicken broth 2 lbs boneless skinless chicken thighs Lime wedges and additional sliced scallions for garnish (optional) Jerk Mixture: 2 tbsp molasses 2 tbsp lime juice 2 tbsp paprika 1 ½ tbsp olive oil 1 ½ tbsp garlic powder 1 ½ tsp allspice 1 tsp ground nutmeg 1 tsp kosher salt ¾ tsp cayenne or to taste ¼ tsp pepper

Directions and total time – 30-60 m

• Prepare corn muffin mix according to package directions, then stir in sliced scallions and minced jalapeno. • Coat the inside of a silicone egg bite mold with nonstick spray • Divide corn muffin batter into the egg bite molds. Tap on the counter to even the batter and release and bubbles. Cover loosely with foil--do not seal. • In a medium bowl, combine the Jerk Mixture ingredients and stir until uniform. Reserve half the jerk mixture and set aside. • Add olive oil to the Instant Pot. Using the display panel select the SAUTE function. • Coat the chicken thighs in the remaining jerk mixture, then brown the chicken on both sides, 3-4 minutes per side. Meat will not be cooked through. Do not crowd the pot--you may have to work in batches. Transfer browned meat to a shallow dish and cover loosely with foil. • Add broth to the pot and deglaze by using a wooden spoon to scrape the brown bits from the bottom of the pot. • Add chicken to the pot in an even layer, then spread remaining jerk mixture on the chicken. • 9. Insert the steam rack and lower the egg bite mold onto the riser using a foil sling. • Turn the pot off by selecting CANCEL, then secure the lid, making sure the vent is closed. • Using the display panel select the MANUAL or PRESSURE COOK function. Use the +/- keys and program the Instant Pot for 10 minutes. • When the time is up, let the pressure naturally release for 5 minutes, then quick-release the remaining pressure. • Serve the chicken with cornbread. Garnish with lime wedges and additional sliced scallions, if desired.

Pumpkin and Bacon Soup
Ingredients for 4 servings:
2 tbsp coconut oil 4 slices no-sugar-added bacon finely chopped and cooked 2 cups grass-fed beef bone broth 2 cups organic pumpkin purée 2 cups full fat coconut milk ½ cup full-fat Cheddar cheese shredded (optional) ½ tsp crushed red pepper ½ tsp kosher salt ½ tsp freshly ground black pepper ½ cup heavy whipping cream

Directions and total time – 15 m
• Add all ingredients to the Instant Pot. Stir and mix thoroughly. • Close the lid, set the pressure release to Sealing, and hit Cancel to stop the current program. Select Manual/Pressure Cook, set the Instant Pot to 10 minutes on low pressure, and let cook. • Once cooked, let the pressure naturally disperse from the Instant Pot for about 10 minutes, then carefully switch the pressure release to Venting. Open the Instant Pot, serve, and enjoy!

Simple Lasagna

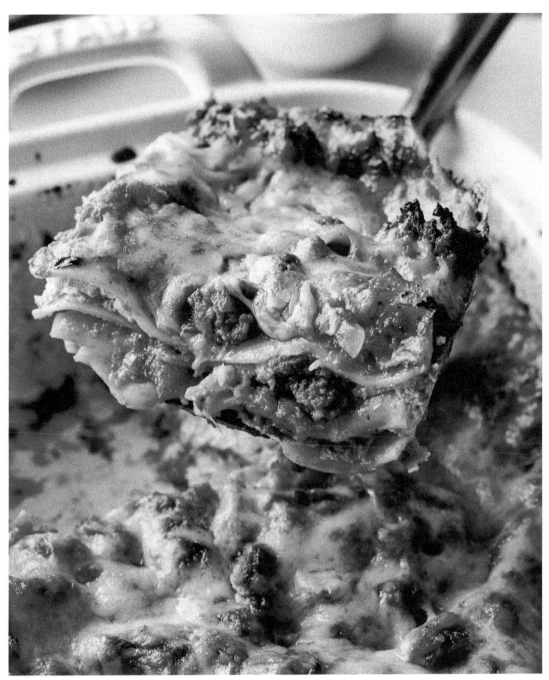

Ingredients for 8 servings:
1 tbsp olive oil 1 tbsp butter 1 small onion chopped 1 tbsp minced Garlic 2 lbs lean ground beef 1 jar pasta sauce 2 cups beef broth ¼ cup red wine 1 cup Water 1 tbsp Italian seasoning 8 oz uncooked lasagna noodles or other pasta. 2 cups shredded mozzarella cheese divided ¼ cup Parmesan cheese 1 cup ricotta cheese
Directions and total time – 30-60 m

• Set Instant Pot to SAUTE. Add the olive oil and butter and allow it to sizzle. Add the onions and garlic cook for 2 minutes. Stir regularly. • Add ground beef and cook until about 4 - 5 minutes, or until no longer pink. Drain grease and return to Instant Pot. • Add pasta sauce, beef broth, wine, water and Italian seasonings. Mix well. • Add pasta. Stir to make sure noodles are covered with the liquid. • Set Instant Pot to MANUAL or PRESSURE COOK on HIGH PRESSURE for 20 minutes. Lock lid and make sure vent is closed. When coking time ends, release pressure and wait for steam to completely stop before opening lid. • Stir in cheese, but reserve about ½ cup mozzarella cheese if you would like to sprinkle a bit on top of the lasagna when you serve it.

Risotto Bolognese
Ingredients for 4-6 servings:
3 slices bacon chopped ½ of an onion finely diced ½ cup carrot diced ½ cup celery diced 1 clove garlic minced 1 cup risotto rice ⅓ cup marsala wine 5 cups beef broth warmed 14.5 oz can diced tomatoes undrained 6 oz cooked sausage crumbles 1 tbsp tomato paste 1 bay leaf ¼ cup freshly grated parmesan 2 tbsp chopped fresh parsley and additional grated parmesan for garnish

Directions and total time – 30-60 m
• Add bacon to the Instant Pot. Using the display panel select the SAUTE function. Cook and stir until bacon is nearly crisp. • Add onion, carrot, celery and garlic to the pot and saute until softened, 4-5 minutes. • Add rice and cook and stir 3 minutes more. • Add wine and broth to the pot and deglaze by using a wooden spoon to scrape the brown bits from the bottom of the pot. • Add diced tomatoes and their juices, sausage crumbles, tomato paste and bay leaf. Stir to incorporate. • Turn the pot off by selecting CANCEL, then secure the lid, making sure the vent is closed. • Using the display panel select the MANUAL or PRESSURE function. Use the +/- keys and program the Instant Pot for 10 minutes. • When the time is up, let the pressure naturally release for 5 minutes, then quick-release the remaining pressure. • Stir to incorporate remaining liquid, returning to SAUTE mode as needed. • Stir in parmesan and adjust seasonings. • Serve hot garnished with chopped fresh parsley and additional grated parmesan.

Shepherd's Pie

Ingredients for 4-6 servings: 1 tablespoon avocado oil or other neutral oil with high smoke point 1 pound ground lamb or beef 1 yellow onion, diced 1 celery stalk, diced 1 large carrot, diced 1 garlic clove, minced 1 ¼ teaspoons kosher salt 1 teaspoon dried thyme ½ teaspoon freshly ground black pepper 1 tablespoon Worcestershire sauce 1 tablespoon tomato paste 1 cup vegetable broth 1 cup frozen peas 4 medium russet potatoes, peeled (about 2 ½ pounds) ½ cup whole milk

Directions and total time – 30-60 m • Select the Sauté setting on the Instant Pot and heat the avocado oil. Add the lamb and sauté, breaking it up with a wooden spoon or spatula, for about 7 minutes, until cooked through and no traces of pink remain. Set a colander in a bowl. Wearing heat-resistant mitts, lift out the inner pot and pour the lamb into the colander, letting it drain. Return the inner pot to the Instant Pot housing. Pressure Cooker Shepherd's Pie - brown the beef or lamb. • Cook the vegetables and stir in the meat: Add the onion, celery, carrot, garlic, and ½ teaspoon of the salt to the pot and sauté for about 4 minutes, until the onion is translucent. Stir in the thyme, pepper, Worcestershire, and tomato paste. Return the lamb to the pot, then add the vegetable broth and peas. • Pressure Cooker Shepherd's Pie - add the vegetables Pressure Cooker Shepherd's Pie - finish cooking the filling. • Add the potatoes: Place a tall steam rack in the pot, making sure all of its legs are resting firmly on the bottom. Place the potatoes in a single layer on the rack. Pressure Cooker Shepherd's Pie - place the cooking rack over the vegetables Pressure Cooker Shepherd's Pie - place the potatoes on top • Pressure cook the filling and the potatoes together: Secure the lid and set the Pressure Release to Sealing. Press the Cancel button to reset the cooking program, then select the Pressure Cook or Manual program and set the cooking time for 15 minutes at high pressure. (The pot will take about 15 minutes to come up to pressure before the cooking program begins.). Pressure Cooker Shepherd's Pie - cook the potatoes and filling • Vent the pressure: When the cooking program ends, perform a quick pressure release by moving the Pressure Release to Venting. • Mash the potatoes: Using tongs, transfer the potatoes to a bowl. Add the milk and remaining ¾ teaspoon salt, then use a potato masher to mash the potatoes until smooth. • Wearing heat-resistant mitts, remove the steam rack from the pot. Stir ½ cup of the mashed potatoes into the lamb mixture in the pot. Pressure Cooker Shepherd's Pie - Remove the cooked potatoes Pressure Cooker Shepherd's Pie - Mash the potatoes Pressure Cooker Shepherd's Pie -

Stir in the mashed potatoes • Assemble the casserole: Transfer the lamb mixture to a broiler-safe 8-inch square baking dish, dollop the mashed potatoes on top, and spread them out with a fork, creating a surface texture. • Broil the casserole: Broil the shepherd's pie in a toaster oven (or a conventional oven) for about 5 minutes, checking often, until the potatoes are lightly browned. • 9 Serve: Spoon the shepherd's pie onto plates and serve immediately.

Rice and Chicken

Ingredients for 4-6 servings: For the sauce: ¼ cup dry sherry ¾ cup chicken broth ½ cup sour cream ¼ cup heavy cream 1 ½ teaspoons Italian seasoning 1 ¼ teaspoons salt ½ teaspoon ground pepper ½ teaspoon paprika For the casserole: 1 tablespoon olive oil 1 medium onion, diced ½ pound crimini mushrooms, sliced 2 cloves garlic, minced 1 ½ pounds (5 to 6) boneless skinless chicken thighs, cut into 1 ½-inch pieces 1 ½ cups long grain white rice To serve: ¼ cup chopped parsley

Directions and total time – 15-30 m • Whisk together the sauce: In a mixing bowl or large liquid measuring cup, whisk together the sherry, chicken broth, sour cream, cream, Italian seasoning, salt, pepper, and paprika. Set aside. • Sauté the vegetables in the pressure cooker: Select the "Sauté" setting on the pressure cooker and heat the oil in the pressure cooker. (If you are using a stovetop pressure cooker, heat the oil over medium heat.) • Add the onion and cook for 4 minutes, until a bit softened but not browned. Add the mushrooms and cook until they begin to wilt and give up their liquid, about 3 more minutes. Stir in the garlic and sauté for 1 more minute. • Add the chicken: Stir in the chicken thighs and let them cook for 5 to 6 minutes, stirring often, until opaque and mostly cooked through (it's fine if they're still a little pink in the middle). • Add the rice and the sauce: Use your spatula to pat the chicken and vegetables down into a fairly even layer. Sprinkle the rice over the top of the chicken in an even layer. Slowly pour the sauce over the rice, taking care not to disturb the layer. Use a spoon to nudge down any grains of rice that are clinging to the sides of the pot, so everything is covered with the cooking liquid. • Pressure cook the chicken and rice: Secure the lid on the pressure cooker. Make sure that the pressure regulator is set to the "Sealing" position. Cancel the "Sauté" program on the pressure cooker, then select the "Manual" or "Pressure Cook" setting. Set the cooking time to 5 minutes at high pressure. (If using a stovetop pressure cooker, the cooking time is the same.). The pressure cooker will take 5 to 10 minutes to come up to pressure before the cooking time begins. • Let the pressure release naturally for at least 10 minutes, then quick-release the pressure by immediately moving the vent from "Sealing" to "Venting." Be careful of the steam! Alternatively, you can let the pot continue to depressurize naturally, which takes about 20 minutes total. The sauce may look a little bit separated when you initially open the pot. Don't worry, it's fine! Just use a fork to gently fluff the rice and incorporate the creamy layer back into the casserole. • Serve the casserole: Spoon the casserole into shallow bowls or onto plates, digging all the way down to the bottom so you get both rice and chicken in each scoop. Sprinkle generously with chopped parsley and serve hot. • Leftovers will keep for about a week and can be warmed in the microwave.

Best Mashed Potatoes
Ingredients for 6-8 servings:

2 ½ teaspoons Chinese Five-Spice Powder 3 to 3 ½ pounds pork shoulder, cut into large chunks (3- to 4-inch pieces) ⅓ cup water ¼ cup hoisin sauce 3 tablespoons soy sauce 3 tablespoons honey 2 tablespoons dry sherry 1 tablespoon cooking oil (I like avocado oil) 5 cloves garlic, minced 2-inch (1-ounce) piece ginger, minced

Directions and total time – 1-2 h

• Sprinkle the spice blend evenly over the pork chunks, making sure to coat them on all sides. • Make the sauce: In a small bowl, whisk together the water, hoisin sauce, soy sauce, honey, and sherry. • Cook the garlic and ginger in the pressure cooker: Select the "Sauté" setting and heat the oil in your electric pressure cooker. Add the garlic and ginger, and sauté until the garlic is fragrant but not yet beginning to brown, 1 to 2 minutes. • Pressure cook the pork: Use a pair of tongs to add the seasoned pieces of pork into the pressure cooker, arranging them in a single layer. Pour the cooking sauce over top. • Secure the lid on the pressure cooker. Make sure that the pressure regulator is set to the "Sealing" position. Cancel the "Sauté" program on the pressure cooker, then select the "Manual" or "Pressure Cook" setting. Set the cooking time to 55 minutes at high pressure. (The pressure cooker will take about 10 minutes to come up to pressure and then the actual cooking time will begin.) • Release the pressure: You can either perform a quick pressure release by immediately moving the vent from "Sealing" to "Venting" (be careful of the steam), or you can let the pot depressurize naturally, which takes about 20 minutes • Separate the pork and cooking liquid. Use tongs to transfer the pork to a large platter or sheet pan. Use heatproof mitts to lift the inner pot out of the pressure cooker, pour the cooking liquid into a fat separator, then pour the liquid back into the pot. (If you don't have a fat separator, let the cooking liquid stand for about 10 minutes until the fat floats to the top, then use a to skim as much fat as possible from the surface.). • Reduce the cooking liquid: Return the pot to the pressure cooker, select the "Sauté" program, and let the cooking liquid come to a rapid simmer. Continue simmering for 10 minutes to reduce the cooking liquid. • While the liquid is reducing, use a pair of forks to shred the pork. • Toss the shredded pork with the reduced liquid: Return the pork to the pot with the reduced cooking liquid and toss to coat the pork evenly. If the pork seems a little dry, add a tablespoon or two of the reserved fat. • Serve the pulled pork with scallions sprinkled over top.

BBQ Baby Back Ribs
Ingredients for 4-6 servings:
2 full racks baby back ribs (3-4 pounds) about ⅓ cup dry rub for pork, store-bought or homemade ¾ cup water ¾ cup apple cider vinegar ½ teaspoon liquid smoke (optional) 2 cups barbecue sauce, favorite store-bought or homemade

Directions and total time – 1-2 h
• Prep the ribs: Working with one rack at a time, use a paring knife to separate the thin transparent membrane on the inside of the ribs. Peel it away from the ribs. It should come off in one big piece. This will make it easier to slice and serve the ribs. • Apply the rub: Rub the ribs well on all sides with dry rub. If possible, cover and let rest in the fridge overnight. • Cook the ribs: In the bottom of your Instant Pot, add some foil balls or a rack to raise the ribs above the liquid. Pour water, vinegar, and liquid smoke (optional) into the Instant Pot. Add ribs, bending them to fit. You should be able to fit two racks of baby back ribs in a 6-quart Instant Pot or pressure cooker. Lock the pressure cooker and cook on high pressure for 30 minutes. Release the pressure naturally for 10 minutes, then vent off remaining pressure. • Broil the ribs: Remove ribs from the Instant Pot and spread them out on a baking sheet. Brush liberally with barbecue sauce and broil on high heat for 5 minutes. Slice ribs and serve with sides and extra sauce. • To reheat leftover ribs, wrap them tightly in foil and heat them in a 350°F oven until heated through, about 15 minutes. You can also grill them for 10-15 minutes over medium heat. Serve with extra sauce!

Potato Salad

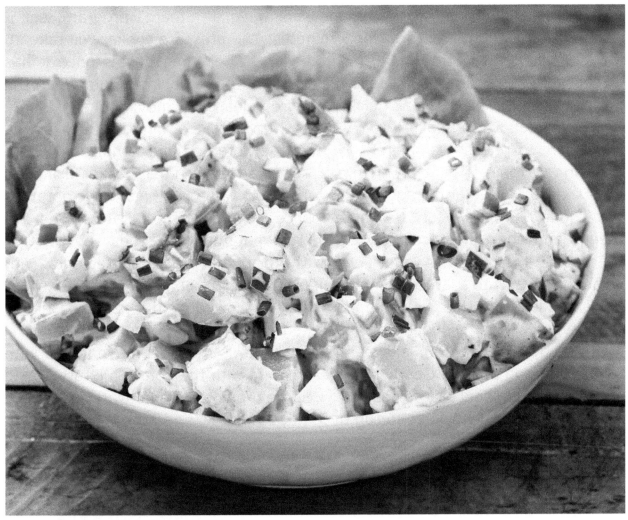

Ingredients for 6-8 servings:

3 or 4 medium Russet or Yukon Gold potatoes (2 to 3 pounds), peeled and quartered if Russets, halved if Yukon Gold 2 large eggs ¼ cup pickle juice from a jar of Kosher dill pickles (plus more to taste) 3 tablespoons finely chopped dill pickles ¼ cup chopped parsley ½ cup chopped red onion 2 stalks celery, chopped 1 or 2 chopped scallions, including the greens 1 medium carrot, peeled and finely chopped ½ red bell pepper, chopped ½ cup mayonnaise 2 teaspoons Dijon mustard ½ teaspoon ground black pepper Salt to taste

Directions and total time – 15-30 m

• Cook the potatoes and eggs in the pressure cooker: Pour a cup of water into a pressure cooker and place a steamer basket inside. Add the quartered potatoes and place the eggs on top. Secure the lid on the pressure cooker.

Make sure that the pressure regulator is set to the "Sealing" position. If you are using an Instant Pot, select the "Steam" program, then adjust the time to 5 minutes. If your pressure does not have a "Steam" program, set it manually to "High Pressure" for 5 minutes. The pressure cooker will take 10 to 15 minutes to come up to full pressure. Cook time begins once it has reached full pressure. • Release the pressure after cooking: Right when the timer goes off, perform a quick pressure release by moving the pressure release knob from "Sealing" to "Venting." It will take a minute or two for the pressure to release completely. • Cool the potatoes and eggs, then chop. Wearing a pair of heat-proof mitts, remove the steamer basket from the pressure cooker. Put the eggs in a bowl of cold water, and leave the potatoes to cool in the basket for 10 minutes. Once cool, cube the potatoes. Peel the eggs and chop them coarsely. Keep the potatoes and eggs separate. • Combine the potatoes and eggs with the other salad ingredients: Put the potatoes into a large mixing bowl. Gently fold in the juice from the Kosher dill pickles. Add the finely chopped pickles followed by the parsley, onions, celery, scallions, chopped hard-boiled eggs, carrots, and red bell pepper. • Mix in the dressing: In a separate small bowl, mix the mayonnaise with mustard and pepper. Gently fold the dressing with the potato mixture. Taste and add additional salt as needed. • Serve the potato salad warm or chilled. The potato salad will keep for up to 3 days in the refrigerator.

Meat for Sandwich
Ingredients for 6-8 servings:
 Boneless Skinless Turkey Breast, 2-3 pounds ½ cup seasoning of choice 2 garlic cloves minced (optional) 1 cup chicken broth
Directions and total time – 30-60 m
• Season the turkey with your seasonings. • Insert the trivet into your liner. • Pour the chicken broth into the pot. • Place the turkey on top of the trivet. • Add minced garlic onto the breast (optional) • Using the manual setting, set the timer to 30 minutes. • Once the timer beeps, release the pressure (quick release). • Check the internal temperature and ensure it is at least 165F • Let the meat cool, and then cut the strings off and slice thinly. If you let it sit in the fridge overnight it will be much easier to slice.

Kale and Tomato Frittata
(Ready in about 10 minutes | Servings 3)
Per serving: 140 Calories; 7.3g Fat; 8.1g Carbs; 11.2g Protein; 2.8g Sugars

Ingredients

5 eggs, whisked 1 cup fresh kale leaves, torn into pieces 1 green bell pepper, seeded and chopped 1 jalapeño pepper, seeded and minced 1 fresh ripe tomato, chopped Sea salt and ground black pepper, to taste 1/2 teaspoon cayenne pepper 2 tablespoons scallions, chopped 1 garlic clove, minced

Directions

Spritz a baking pan that fits inside your Instant Pot with a nonstick cooking spray. Thoroughly combine all ingredients and spoon the mixture into the prepared baking pan. Cover with a sheet of foil. Add 1 cup of water and a metal trivet to the Instant Pot. Lower the baking pan onto the trivet. Secure the lid. Choose "Manual" mode and Low pressure; cook for 6 minutes. Once cooking is complete, use a natural pressure release; carefully remove the lid. Serve warm. Bon appétit!

Mom's Cheesy Soup
(Ready in about 25 minutes | Servings 4
Per serving: 530 Calories; 37.6g Fat; 4.2g Carbs; 43.1g Protein; 1.9g Sugars

Ingredients

2 tablespoons butter, melted 1/2 cup leeks, chopped 2 chicken breasts, trimmed and cut into bite-sized chunks 1 carrot, chopped 1 celery stalk, chopped 1/2 teaspoon granulated garlic 1 teaspoon basil 1/2 teaspoon oregano 1/2 teaspoon dill weed 4 ½ cups vegetable stock 3 ounces heavy cream 3/4 cup Cheddar cheese, shredded 1 heaping tablespoon fresh parsley, roughly chopped

Directions

Press the "Sauté" button to heat up your Instant Pot. Now, melt the butter and cook the leeks until tender and fragrant. Add the chicken, carrot, celery, garlic, basil, oregano, dill, and stock. Secure the lid. Choose "Manual" mode and High pressure; cook for 17 minutes. Once cooking is complete, use a natural pressure release; carefully remove the lid. Add cream and cheese, stir, and press the "Sauté" button one more time. Now, cook the soup for a couple of minutes longer or until thoroughly heated. Serve in individual bowls, garnished with fresh parsley. Bon appétit!

Golden Cheddar Muffins with Chard
(Ready in about 10 minutes | Servings 4)
Per serving: 207 Calories; 14.8g Fat; 4.9g Carbs; 13.4g Protein; 2.7g Sugars
Ingredients
6 eggs 4 tablespoons double cream Sea salt and ground black pepper, to taste 1 cup Swiss chard, chopped 1 red bell pepper, chopped 1/2 cup white onion, chopped 1/2 cup Cheddar cheese, grated
Directions
Begin by adding 1 cup of water and a metal rack to the Instant Pot. Mix all of the above ingredients. Then, fill silicone muffin cups about 2/3 full. Then, place muffin cups on the rack. Secure the lid. Choose "Manual" mode and High pressure; cook for 7 minutes. Once cooking is complete, use a natural pressure release; carefully remove the lid. Enjoy!

The Best Homemade Cheese Ever
(Ready in about 1 hour | Servings 14)
Per serving: 134 Calories; 6.9g Fat; 9.1g Carbs; 6.8g Protein; 10.9g Sugars

Ingredients

3 quarts milk 1/2 cup distilled vinegar 1/2 cup heavy cream 1 teaspoon kosher salt

Directions

Add milk to your Instant Pot and secure the lid. Choose "Yogurt" mode; now, press the "Adjust" button until you see the word "Boil". Whisk a few times during the cooking time. Use a food thermometer to read temperature; 180 degrees is fine. Gradually whisk in the vinegar. Turn off the Instant Pot. Cover with the lid; now, allow it to sit for 40 minutes. Stir in the cream and salt. Pour the cheese into a colander lined with a tea towel; allow it to sit and drain for 15 minutes. Afterwards, squeeze it as dry as possible and transfer to your refrigerator. Enjoy!

Bacon and Pepper Casserole with Goat Cheese

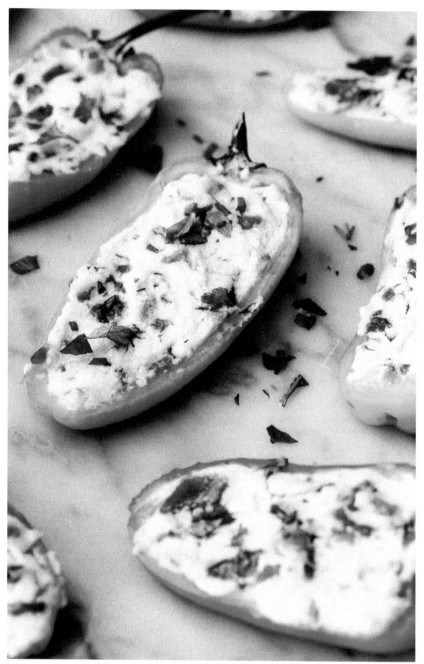

(Ready in about 30 minutes | Servings 4)
 Per serving: 494 Calories; 41.3g Fat; 7.8g Carbs; 25.5g Protein; 3.5g Sugars

Ingredients

6 ounces bacon, chopped 1 green bell pepper, seeded and chopped 1 orange bell pepper, seeded and chopped 1 Cascabella chili pepper, seeded and minced

5 eggs 3/4 cup heavy cream 6 ounces goat cheese, crumbled Sea salt and ground black pepper, to your liking

Directions

Add 1 cup of water and a metal trivet to the Instant Pot. Lower the baking pan onto the trivet. Spritz a baking dish that fits inside your Instant Pot with a nonstick cooking spray. Place the bacon on the bottom of the dish. Add the peppers on the top. In a mixing bowl, thoroughly combine the eggs, heavy cream, goat cheese, salt, and black pepper. Spoon this mixture over the top. Secure the lid. Choose "Manual" mode and High pressure; cook for 15 minutes. Once cooking is complete, use a natural pressure release; carefully remove the lid. Allow your frittata to cool for 10 minutes before slicing and serving. Bon appétit!

Zingy Habanero Eggs

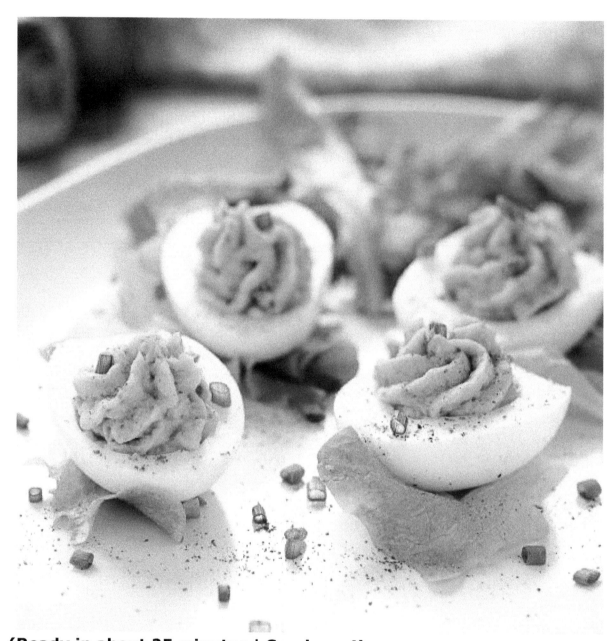

(Ready in about 25 minutes | Servings 4)
Per serving: 338 Calories; 25.7g Fat; 5.8g Carbs; 19.8g Protein; 2.8g Sugars
Ingredients
8 eggs 2 teaspoons habanero chili pepper, minced 1 teaspoon cumin seeds 1/4 cup sour cream 1/4 cup mayonnaise 1 teaspoon stone-ground mustard 1/2 teaspoon cayenne pepper Sea salt and freshly ground black pepper, to taste
Directions

Pour 1 cup of water into the Instant Pot; add a steamer basket to the bottom. Arrange the eggs in the steamer basket. Secure the lid. Choose "Manual" mode and High pressure; cook for 5 minutes. Once cooking is complete, use a natural pressure release; carefully remove the lid. Allow the eggs to cool for 15 minutes. Peel the eggs and separate egg whites from yolks. Press the "Sauté" button to heat up your Instant Pot; heat the oil. Now, sauté habanero chili pepper and cumin seeds until they are fragrant. Add the reserved egg yolks to the pepper mixture. Stir in sour cream, mayonnaise, mustard, cayenne pepper, salt, and black pepper. Now, stuff the egg whites with this mixture. Bon appétit!

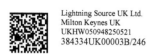

9 781008 958494